Skill Checklists for

Fundamentals of Nursing

THE ART AND SCIENCE OF PERSON-CENTERED CARE

Skill Checklists for

Fundamentals of Nursing

THE ART AND SCIENCE OF PERSON-CENTERED CARE

NINTH EDITION

Carol Taylor, PhD, MSN, RN
Professor of Nursing
Georgetown University School of Nursing and Health Studies
Washington, DC

Pamela Lynn, EdD, MSN, RN
Assistant Professor
Frances M. Maguire School of Nursing and Health Professions
Gwynedd Mercy University
Gwynedd Valley, Pennsylvania

Jennifer L. Bartlett, PhD, RN-BC, CNE, CHSE
Assistant Professor
Georgia Baptist College of Nursing of Mercer University
Atlanta, Georgia

 Wolters Kluwer

Philadelphia • Baltimore • New York • London
Buenos Aires • Hong Kong • Sydney • Tokyo

Vice President and Publisher: Julie K. Stegman
Acquisitions Editor: Natasha McIntyre
Director of Product Development: Jennifer K. Forestieri
Editorial Coordinator: Emily Buccieri
Marketing Manager: Brittany Clements
Production Project Manager: Linda Van Pelt
Design Coordinator: Holly Reid McLaughlin
Illustration Coordinator: Jennifer Clements
Manufacturing Coordinator: Karin Duffield
Prepress Vendor: Aptara, Inc.

9th Edition

9 8 7 6 5 4 3 2 1

Printed in China

ISBN: 9781975102449

Introduction

Developing clinical competency is an important challenge for each fundamentals nursing student. To facilitate the mastery of nursing skills, we are happy to provide skill checklists for each skill included in *Fundamentals of Nursing: The Art and Science of Person-Centered Care,* Ninth Edition. Students can use the checklists to facilitate self-evaluation, and faculty will find them useful in measuring and recording student performance. Three-hole-punched and perforated, these checklists can be easily reproduced and brought to the simulation laboratory or clinical area.

The checklists follow each step of the skill to provide a complete evaluative tool. They are designed to record an evaluation of each step of the procedure.

- Checkmark in the "Excellent" column denotes mastering the procedure.
- Checkmark in the "Satisfactory" column indicates use of the recommended technique.
- Checkmark in the "Needs Practice" column indicates use of some but not all of each recommended technique.

The Comments section allows you to highlight suggestions that will improve skills. Space is available at the top of each checklist to record a final pass/fail evaluation, date, and the signature of the student and evaluating faculty member.

Faculty who adopt this book will also find on thePoint website at http://thepoint.lww.com/TaylorCklst9e a *Master Skills Competency Checklist* to aid in record keeping.

List of Skills by Chapter

List of Skills in Alphabetical Order

Skills Checklist to Accompany Fundamentals of Nursing:
The Art and Science of Person-Centered Care, 9th edition

Name _____ Date _____

Unit _____ Position _____

Instructor/Evaluator: _____ Position _____

Excellent	Satisfactory	Needs Practice	SKILL 24-1 **Performing Hand Hygiene Using Soap and Water (Handwashing)**	
			Goal: The hands are free of visible soiling and transient microorganisms are eliminated.	**Comments**
___	___	___	1. Gather the necessary supplies. Stand in front of the sink. Do not allow your clothing to touch the sink during the washing procedure.	
___	___	___	2. Remove jewelry, if possible, and secure in a safe place. A plain wedding band may remain in place.	
___	___	___	3. Turn on water and adjust force. Regulate the temperature until the water is warm.	
___	___	___	4. Wet the hands and wrist area. Keep hands lower than elbows to allow water to flow toward fingertips.	
___	___	___	5. Use about 1 teaspoon liquid soap from dispenser or rinse bar of soap and lather thoroughly. Cover all areas of hands with the soap product. If using bar soap, rinse soap bar again and return to soap rack without touching the rack.	
___	___	___	6. With firm rubbing and circular motions, wash the palms and backs of the hands, each finger, the areas between the fingers, and the knuckles, wrists, and forearms. *Wash at least 1 in above area of contamination.* If hands are not visibly soiled, wash to 1 in above the wrists.	
___	___	___	7. Continue this friction motion for at least 20 seconds.	
___	___	___	8. Use fingernails of the opposite hand or a clean orangewood stick to clean under fingernails.	
___	___	___	9. Rinse thoroughly with water flowing toward fingertips.	
___	___	___	10. Pat hands dry with a paper towel, beginning with the fingers and moving upward toward forearms, and discard it immediately. Use another clean towel to turn off the faucet. Discard towel immediately without touching other clean hand.	
___	___	___	11. Use oil-free lotion on hands, if desired.	

Skills Checklist to Accompany Fundamentals of Nursing:
The Art and Science of Person-Centered Care, 9th edition

Name _____ Date _____

Unit _____ Position _____

Instructor/Evaluator: _____ Position _____

Excellent	Satisfactory	Needs Practice	SKILL 24-2 **Using Personal Protective Equipment (PPE)**

Goal: The transmission of microorganisms is prevented.   **Comments**

Excellent	Satisfactory	Needs Practice	
——	——	——	1. Check medical record and nursing care plan for type of precautions and review precautions in infection control manual.
——	——	——	2. Plan nursing activities before entering patient's room.
——	——	——	3. Provide instruction about precautions to patient, family members, and visitors.
——	——	——	4. Perform hand hygiene.
——	——	——	5. Put on gown, mask, protective eyewear, and gloves based on the type of exposure anticipated and category of isolation precautions.
——	——	——	a. Put on the gown, with the opening in the back. Tie gown securely at neck and waist.
——	——	——	b. Put on the mask or respirator over your nose, mouth, and chin. Secure ties or elastic bands at the middle of the head and neck. If respirator is used, perform a fit check. Inhale; the respirator should collapse. Exhale; air should not leak out.
——	——	——	c. Put on goggles. Place over eyes and adjust to fit. Alternately, a face shield could be used to take the place of the mask and goggles.
——	——	——	d. Put on clean disposable gloves. Extend gloves to cover the cuffs of the gown.
——	——	——	6. Identify the patient. Explain the procedure to the patient. Continue with patient care as appropriate.

Excellent	Satisfactory	Needs Practice		Comments

Remove PPE

7. Remove PPE: Except for respirator, remove PPE at the doorway or in an anteroom. ***Remove respirator after leaving the patient's room and closing the door.***

   a. If impervious gown has been tied in front of the body at the waistline, untie waist strings before removing gloves.

   b. Grasp the outside of one glove with the opposite gloved hand and peel off, turning the glove inside out as you pull it off. Hold the removed glove in the remaining gloved hand.

   c. Slide fingers of ungloved hand under the remaining glove at the wrist, **taking care not to touch the outer surface of the glove.**

   d. Peel off the glove over the first glove, containing the one glove inside the other. Discard in appropriate container.

   e. To remove the goggles or face shield: Handle by the headband or earpieces. Lift away from the face. Place in designated receptacle for reprocessing or in an appropriate waste container.

   f. To remove gown: Unfasten ties, if at the neck and back. Allow the gown to fall away from shoulders. ***Touching only the inside of the gown,*** pull away from the torso. Keeping hands on the inner surface of the gown, pull gown from arms. Turn gown inside out. Fold or roll into a bundle and discard.

   g. To remove mask or respirator: Grasp the neck ties or elastic, then top ties or elastic and remove. ***Take care to avoid touching front of mask or respirator.*** Discard in waste container. If using a respirator, save for future use in the designated area.

8. Perform hand hygiene immediately after removing all PPE.

4

Skills Checklist to Accompany Fundamentals of Nursing:
The Art and Science of Person-Centered Care, 9th edition

Name _____ Date _____

Unit _____ Position _____

Instructor/Evaluator: _____ Position _____

Excellent	Satisfactory	Needs Practice	SKILL 24-3 **Preparing a Sterile Field and Adding Sterile Items to a Sterile Field**	Comments
			Goal: The sterile field is created without contamination and the patient remains free of exposure to potential infection-causing microorganisms.	
___	___	___	1. Perform hand hygiene and put on PPE, if indicated.	
___	___	___	2. Identify the patient. Explain the procedure to the patient.	
			Preparing a Sterile Field	
___	___	___	3. Check that the packaged kit or tray is dry and unopened. Also note expiration date, making sure that the date is still valid.	
___	___	___	4. Select a work area that is waist level or higher.	
___	___	___	5. Open the outside cover of the package and remove the kit or tray. Place in the center of the work surface, with the topmost flap positioned on the far side of the package. Discard outside cover.	
			For a Prepackaged Sterile Drape	
___	___	___	a. Open the outer covering of the drape. Remove sterile drape, lifting it carefully by its corners. Hold away from body and above the waist and work surface.	
___	___	___	b. Continue to hold only by the corners. Allow the drape to unfold, away from your body and any other surface.	
___	___	___	c. Position the drape on the work surface with the moisture-proof side down. This would be the shiny or blue side. Avoid touching any other surface or object with the drape. If any portion of the drape hangs off the work surface, that part of the drape is considered contaminated.	
			For a Commercially Prepared Kit or Tray	
___	___	___	a. Open the outside cover of the package and remove the kit or tray. Place in the center of the work surface, with the topmost flap positioned on the far side of the package. Discard outside cover.	
___	___	___	b. Reach around the package and grasp the outer surface of the end of the topmost flap, holding no more than 1 in from the border of the flap. Pull open away from the body, keeping the arm outstretched and away from the inside of the wrapper. Allow the wrapper to lie flat on the work surface.	

Excellent	Satisfactory	Needs Practice	

Preparing a Sterile Field and Adding
Sterile Items to a Sterile Field (Continued)

Comments

— — —   c. Reach around the package and grasp the outer surface of the first side flap, holding no more than 1 in from the border of the flap. Pull open to the side of the package, keeping the arm outstretched and away from the inside of the wrapper. Allow the wrapper to lie flat on the work surface.

— — —   d. Reach around the package and grasp the outer surface of the remaining side flap, holding no more than 1 in from the border of the flap. Pull open to the side of the package, keeping the arm outstretched and away from the inside of the wrapper. Allow the wrapper to lie flat on the work surface.

— — —   e. Stand away from the package and work surface. Grasp the outer surface of the remaining flap closest to the body, holding not more than 1 in from the border of the flap. Pull the flap back toward the body, keeping arm outstretched and away from the inside of the wrapper. Keep this hand in place. Use other hand to grasp the wrapper on the underside (the side that is down to the work surface). Position the wrapper so that when flat, edges are on the work surface, and do not hang down over sides of work surface. Allow the wrapper to lie flat on the work surface.

— — —   f. The outer wrapper of the package has become a sterile field with the packaged supplies in the center. Do not touch or reach over the sterile field. Place additional sterile items on field as needed. Continue with the procedure as indicated.

Adding Items to a Sterile Field

— — —   6. Place additional sterile items on field as needed.

To Add a Facility-Wrapped and Sterilized Item

— — —   a. Hold facility-wrapped item in the dominant hand, with top flap opening away from the body. With other hand, reach around the package and unfold top flap and both sides.

— — —   b. Keep a secure hold on the item through the wrapper with the dominant hand. Grasp the remaining flap of the wrapper closest to the body, taking care not to touch the inner surface of the wrapper or the item. Pull the flap back toward the wrist, so the wrapper covers the hand and wrist.

Preparing a Sterile Field and Adding Sterile Items to a Sterile Field *(Continued)*

Excellent	Satisfactory	Needs Practice		Comments

—— —— ——		c. Grasp all the corners of the wrapper together with the nondominant hand and pull back toward wrist, covering hand and wrist. Hold in place.	
—— —— ——		d. Hold the item 6 in above the surface of the sterile field and drop onto the field. Be careful to avoid touching the surface or other items or dropping any item onto the 1-in border.	

To Add a Commercially Wrapped and Sterilized Item

—— —— ——		a. Hold package in one hand. Pull back top cover with other hand. Alternately, carefully peel the edges apart using both hands.	
—— —— ——		b. After top cover or edges are partially separated, hold the item 6 in above the surface of the sterile field. Continue opening the package and drop the item onto the field. *Be careful to avoid touching the surface or other items or dropping an item onto the 1-in border.*	
—— —— ——		c. Discard wrapper.	

To Add a Sterile Solution

—— —— ——		a. Obtain appropriate solution and check expiration date.	
—— —— ——		b. Open solution container according to directions and *place cap on table away from the field with edges up.*	
—— —— ——		c. Hold bottle outside the edge of the sterile field with the label side facing the palm of your hand and prepare to pour from a height of 4 to 6 in (10 to 15 cm). *Never touch the tip of the bottle to the sterile container or field.*	
—— —— ——		d. Pour required amount of solution steadily into sterile container previously added to the sterile field and positioned at side of sterile field or onto dressings. *Avoid splashing any liquid.*	
—— —— ——		e. Touch only the outside of the lid when recapping. Label solution with date and time of opening.	
—— —— ——		7. Continue with procedure as indicated.	
—— —— ——		8. When procedure is completed, remove PPE, if used. Perform hand hygiene.	

Skills Checklist to Accompany Fundamentals of Nursing:
The Art and Science of Person-Centered Care, 9th edition

Name _____ Date _____

Unit _____ Position _____

Instructor/Evaluator: _____ Position _____

Excellent	Satisfactory	Needs Practice	SKILL 24-4 **Putting on Sterile Gloves and Removing Soiled Gloves**

SKILL 24-4

Putting on Sterile Gloves and Removing Soiled Gloves

Goal: The gloves are applied and removed without contamination.   **Comments**

Excellent	Satisfactory	Needs Practice		Comments
____	____	____	1. Perform hand hygiene and put on PPE, if indicated.	
____	____	____	2. Identify the patient. Explain the procedure to the patient.	
____	____	____	3. Check that the sterile glove package is dry and unopened. Also note expiration date, making sure that the date is still valid.	
____	____	____	4. Place sterile glove package on clean, dry surface at or above your waist.	
____	____	____	5. Open the outside wrapper by carefully peeling the top layer back. Remove inner package, handling only the outside of it.	
____	____	____	6. Place the inner package on the work surface with the side labeled "cuff end" closest to the body.	
____	____	____	7. Carefully open the inner package. Fold open the top flap, then the bottom and sides. *Do not touch the inner surface of the package or the gloves.*	
____	____	____	8. With the thumb and forefinger of the nondominant hand, grasp the folded cuff of the glove for the dominant hand, touching only the exposed inside of the glove.	
____	____	____	9. Keeping the hands above the waistline, lift and hold the glove up and off the inner package with fingers down. *Do not let it touch any unsterile object.*	
____	____	____	10. Carefully insert dominant hand palm up into glove and pull glove on. Leave the cuff folded until the opposite hand is gloved.	
____	____	____	11. Hold the thumb of the gloved hand outward. Place the fingers of the gloved hand inside the cuff of the remaining glove. Lift it from the wrapper, taking care not to touch anything with the gloves or hands.	
____	____	____	12. Carefully insert nondominant hand into glove. Pull the glove on, taking care that the skin does not touch any of the outer surfaces of the gloves.	

Putting on Sterile Gloves and
Removing Soiled Gloves *(Continued)*

Excellent	Satisfactory	Needs Practice		Comments
—	—	—	13. *Slide the fingers of one hand under the cuff of the other and fully extend the cuff down the arm, touching only the sterile outside of the glove. Repeat for the remaining hand.*	
—	—	—	14. Adjust gloves on both hands if necessary, *touching only sterile areas with other sterile areas.*	
—	—	—	15. Continue with procedure as indicated.	
			Removing Soiled Gloves	
—	—	—	16. Use dominant hand to grasp the opposite glove *near cuff end on the outside exposed area.* Remove it by pulling it off, inverting it as it is pulled, keeping the contaminated area on the inside. Hold the removed glove in the remaining gloved hand.	
—	—	—	17. Slide fingers of ungloved hand between the remaining glove and the wrist. *Take care to avoid touching the outside surface of the glove.* Remove it by pulling it off, inverting it as it is pulled, keeping the contaminated area on the inside, and securing the first glove inside the second.	
—	—	—	18. Discard gloves in appropriate container. Remove additional PPE, if used. Perform hand hygiene.	

Skills Checklist to Accompany Fundamentals of Nursing:
The Art and Science of Person-Centered Care, 9th edition

Name _____   Date _____

Unit _____   Position _____

Instructor/Evaluator: _____   Position _____

Excellent	Satisfactory	Needs Practice	SKILL 25-1 **Assessing Body Temperature**	Comments
			Goal: The patient's temperature is assessed accurately without injury and the patient experiences only minimal discomfort.	
___	___	___	1. Check the medical order or nursing care plan for frequency of measurement and route. More frequent temperature measurement may be appropriate based on nursing judgment.	
___	___	___	2. Perform hand hygiene and put on PPE, if indicated.	
___	___	___	3. Identify the patient.	
___	___	___	4. Close the curtains around the bed and close the door to the room, if possible. Discuss the procedure with the patient and assess the patient's ability to assist with the procedure.	
___	___	___	5. Assemble equipment on the overbed table within reach.	
___	___	___	6. Ensure that the electronic or digital thermometer is in working condition.	
___	___	___	7. Put on gloves, if indicated.	
___	___	___	8. Select the appropriate site based on assessment data.	
___	___	___	9. Follow the steps as outlined below for the appropriate type of thermometer.	
___	___	___	10. When measurement is completed, remove gloves, if worn. Remove additional PPE, if used. Perform hand hygiene.	
			Measuring an Oral Temperature	
___	___	___	11. Remove the electronic unit from the charging unit, and remove the probe from within the recording unit.	
___	___	___	12. Cover thermometer probe with disposable probe cover and slide it on until it snaps into place.	
___	___	___	13. *Place the probe beneath the patient's tongue in the posterior sublingual pocket. Ask the patient to close his or her lips around the probe.*	
___	___	___	14. Continue to hold the probe until you hear a beep. Note the temperature reading.	
___	___	___	15. Remove the probe from the patient's mouth. Dispose of the probe cover by holding the probe over an appropriate receptacle and pressing the probe-release button.	

Excellent	Satisfactory	Needs Practice	SKILL 25-1 **Assessing Body Temperature** *(Continued)*	
				Comments
——	——	——	16. Return the thermometer probe to the storage place within the unit. Return the electronic unit to the charging unit, if appropriate.	
			Measuring a Tympanic Membrane Temperature	
——	——	——	17. If necessary, push the "ON" button and wait for the "ready" signal on the unit.	
——	——	——	18. Attach the disposable cover onto the tympanic probe.	
——	——	——	19. *Insert the probe snugly into the external ear using gentle but firm pressure, angling the thermometer toward the patient's jaw line. Pull the pinna up and back to straighten the ear canal in an adult.*	
——	——	——	20. Activate the unit by pushing the trigger button. The reading is immediate (usually within 2 seconds). Note the reading.	
——	——	——	21. Discard the probe cover in an appropriate receptacle by pushing the probe-release button or use the rim of cover to remove it from the probe. Replace the thermometer in its charger, if necessary.	
			Measuring Temporal Artery Temperature	
——	——	——	22. Brush the patient's hair aside if it is covering the temporal artery area.	
——	——	——	23. Apply a probe cover.	
——	——	——	24. Hold the thermometer like a remote control device, with your thumb on the red "ON" button. Place the probe flush on the center of the forehead, with the body of the instrument sideways (not straight up and down) so that it is not in the patient's face.	
——	——	——	25. Depress the "ON" button. Keep the button depressed throughout the measurement.	
——	——	——	26. Slowly slide the probe straight across the forehead, midline, to the hairline. The thermometer will click; fast clicking indicates a rise to a higher temperature, slow clicking indicates that the instrument is still scanning, but not finding any higher temperature.	
——	——	——	27. If required, based on specific thermometer in use, brush hair aside if it is covering the ear, exposing the area of the neck under the ear lobe. Lift the probe from the forehead and touch on the neck just behind the ear lobe, in the depression just below the mastoid.	

Assessing Body Temperature *(Continued)*

Excellent	Satisfactory	Needs Practice		Comments

28. Release the button and read the thermometer measurement.

29. Hold the thermometer over a waste receptacle. Gently push the probe cover with your thumb against the proximal edge to dispose of the probe cover.

30. The instrument will automatically turn off in 30 seconds, or press and release the power button.

Measuring Axillary Temperature

31. Move the patient's clothing to expose only the axilla.

32. Remove the probe from the recording unit of the electronic thermometer. Place a disposable probe cover on by sliding it on and snapping it securely.

33. *Place the end of the probe in the center of the axilla. Have the patient bring the arm down and close to the body.*

34. Hold the probe in place until you hear a beep, and then carefully remove the probe. Note the temperature reading.

35. Cover the patient and help him or her to a position of comfort.

36. Dispose of the probe cover by holding the probe over an appropriate waste receptacle and pushing the release button.

37. Place the bed in the lowest position and elevate rails, as needed. Leave the patient clean and comfortable.

38. Return the electronic thermometer to the charging unit.

Measuring Rectal Temperature

39. Adjust the bed to a comfortable working height, usually elbow height of the caregiver (VHACEOSH, 2016). Put on nonsterile gloves.

40. Assist the patient to a side-lying position. Pull back the covers sufficiently to expose only the buttocks.

41. Remove the rectal probe from within the recording unit of the electronic thermometer. Cover the probe with a disposable probe cover and slide it until it snaps in place.

42. *Lubricate about 1 in of the probe with a water-soluble lubricant.*

43. Reassure the patient. Separate the buttocks until the anal sphincter is clearly visible.

Assessing Body Temperature *(Continued)*

Excellent	Satisfactory	Needs Practice		Comments
——	——	——	44. *Insert the thermometer probe into the anus about 1.5 in in an adult or no more than 1 in in a child.*	
——	——	——	45. Hold the probe in place until you hear a beep, then carefully remove the probe. Note the temperature reading on the display.	
——	——	——	46. Dispose of the probe cover by holding the probe over an appropriate waste receptacle and pressing the release button.	
——	——	——	47. Using toilet tissue, wipe the anus of any feces or excess lubricant. Dispose of the toilet tissue. Remove gloves and discard them.	
——	——	——	48. Cover the patient and help him or her to a position of comfort.	
——	——	——	49. Place the bed in the lowest position; elevate rails as needed.	
——	——	——	50. Perform hand hygiene.	
——	——	——	51. Return the thermometer to the charging unit.	

Skills Checklist to Accompany Fundamentals of Nursing:
The Art and Science of Person-Centered Care, 9th edition

Name _____ Date _____

Unit _____ Position _____

Instructor/Evaluator: _____ Position _____

Excellent	Satisfactory	Needs Practice	SKILL 25-2 **Assessing a Peripheral Pulse by Palpation**	Comments
			Goal: The patient's pulse is assessed accurately without injury and the patient experiences only minimal discomfort.	
___	___	___	1. Check medical order or nursing care plan for frequency of pulse assessment. More frequent pulse measurement may be appropriate based on nursing judgment.	
___	___	___	2. Perform hand hygiene and put on PPE, if indicated.	
___	___	___	3. Identify the patient.	
___	___	___	4. Close the curtains around the bed and close the door to the room, if possible. Discuss the procedure with the patient and assess the patient's ability to assist with the procedure.	
___	___	___	5. Put on gloves, if indicated.	
___	___	___	6. Select the appropriate peripheral site based on assessment data.	
___	___	___	7. Move the patient's clothing to expose only the site chosen.	
___	___	___	8. Place your first, second, and third fingers over the artery. Place your fingers over the artery so that the ends of your fingers are flat against the patient's skin when palpating peripheral pulses. Do not press with the tip of the fingers only. *Lightly compress the artery so pulsations can be felt and counted.*	
___	___	___	9. Using a watch with a second hand, count the number of pulsations felt for 30 seconds. Multiply this number by 2 to calculate the rate for 1 minute. *If the rate, rhythm, or amplitude of the pulse is abnormal in any way, palpate and count the pulse for 1 minute.*	
___	___	___	10. Note the rhythm and amplitude of the pulse.	
___	___	___	11. When measurement is completed, remove gloves, if worn. Cover the patient and help him or her to a position of comfort.	
___	___	___	12. Remove additional PPE, if used. Perform hand hygiene.	

Skills Checklist to Accompany Fundamentals of Nursing:
The Art and Science of Person-Centered Care, 9th edition

Name _____ Date _____

Unit _____ Position _____

Instructor/Evaluator: _____ Position _____

SKILL 25-3

Assessing Respiration

Excellent	Satisfactory	Needs Practice	**Goal:** The patient's respirations are assessed accurately without injury and the patient experiences only minimal discomfort.	Comments
——	——	——	1. *While your fingers are still in place for the pulse measurement, after counting the pulse rate, observe the patient's respirations.*	
——	——	——	2. Note the rise and fall of the patient's chest.	
——	——	——	3. Using a watch with a second hand, count the number of respirations for 30 seconds. Multiply this number by 2 to calculate the respiratory rate per minute.	
——	——	——	4. *If respirations are abnormal in any way, count the respirations for at least 1 full minute.*	
——	——	——	5. Note the depth and rhythm of the respirations.	
——	——	——	6. When measurement is completed, remove gloves, if worn. Cover the patient and help him or her to a position of comfort.	
——	——	——	7. Remove additional PPE, if used. Perform hand hygiene.	

Skills Checklist to Accompany Fundamentals of Nursing:
The Art and Science of Person-Centered Care, 9th edition

Name _____ Date _____

Unit _____ Position _____

Instructor/Evaluator: _____ Position _____

SKILL 25-4

Assessing Blood Pressure by Auscultation

Excellent	Satisfactory	Needs Practice	**Goal:** The patient's blood pressure is measured accurately with minimal discomfort to the patient.	Comments
――	――	――	1. Check the medical order or nursing care plan for frequency of blood pressure measurement. More frequent measurement may be appropriate based on nursing judgment.	
――	――	――	2. Perform hand hygiene and put on PPE, if indicated.	
――	――	――	3. Identify the patient.	
――	――	――	4. Close the curtains around the bed and close the door to the room, if possible. Discuss the procedure with the patient and assess patient's ability to assist with the procedure. Validate that the patient has relaxed for several minutes.	
――	――	――	5. Put on gloves, if indicated.	
――	――	――	6. Select the appropriate arm for application of the cuff.	
――	――	――	7. Have the patient assume a comfortable lying or sitting position with the forearm supported at the level of the heart and the palm of the hand upward. If the measurement is taken in the supine position, support the arm with a pillow. In the sitting position, support the arm yourself or by using the bedside table. If the patient is sitting, have the patient sit back in the chair so that the chair supports his or her back. In addition, make sure the patient keeps the legs uncrossed.	
――	――	――	8. Expose the brachial artery by removing garments or move a sleeve if it is not too tight, above the area where the cuff will be placed.	
――	――	――	9. Palpate the location of the brachial artery. *Center the bladder of the cuff over the brachial artery, about midway on the arm, so that the lower edge of the cuff is about 2.5 to 5 cm (1 to 2 in) above the inner aspect of the elbow. Line up the artery marking on the cuff with the patient's brachial artery.* The tubing should extend from the edge of the cuff nearer the patient's elbow.	
――	――	――	10. Wrap the cuff around the arm smoothly and snugly, and fasten it. Do not allow any clothing to interfere with the proper placement of the cuff.	
――	――	――	11. Check that the needle on the aneroid gauge is within the zero mark. If using a mercury manometer, check to see that the manometer is in the vertical position and that the mercury is within the zero level with the gauge at eye level.	

SKILL 25-4

Assessing Blood Pressure
by Auscultation *(Continued)*

Excellent	Satisfactory	Needs Practice		Comments

Estimating Systolic Pressure

—— —— —— 12. Palpate the pulse at the brachial or radial artery by pressing gently with the fingertips.

—— —— —— 13. Tighten the screw valve on the air pump.

—— —— —— 14. *Inflate the cuff while continuing to palpate the artery. Note the point on the gauge where the pulse disappears.*

—— —— —— 15. Deflate the cuff and wait 1 minute.

Obtaining Blood Pressure Measurement

—— —— —— 16. Assume a position that is no more than 3 ft away from the gauge.

—— —— —— 17. Place the stethoscope earpieces in your ears. Direct the earpieces forward into the canal and not against the ear itself.

—— —— —— 18. Place the bell or diaphragm of the stethoscope firmly but with as little pressure as possible over the brachial artery. Do not allow the stethoscope to touch clothing or the cuff.

—— —— —— 19. Pump the pressure 30 mm Hg above the point at which the systolic pressure was palpated and estimated. Open the valve on the manometer and allow air to escape slowly (allowing the gauge to drop 2 to 3 mm per second).

—— —— —— 20. *Note the point on the gauge at which the first faint, but clear, sound appears that slowly increases in intensity. Note this number as the systolic pressure. Read the pressure to the closest 2 mm Hg.*

—— —— —— 21. Do not reinflate the cuff once the air is being released to recheck the systolic pressure reading.

—— —— —— 22. *Note the point at which the sound completely disappears. Note this number as the diastolic pressure. Read the pressure to the closest 2 mm Hg.*

—— —— —— 23. Allow the remaining air to escape quickly. Repeat any suspicious reading, but wait at least 1 minute. Deflate the cuff completely between attempts to check the blood pressure.

—— —— —— 24. When measurement is completed, remove the cuff. Remove gloves, if worn. Cover the patient and help him or her to a position of comfort.

—— —— —— 25. Clean the bell or diaphragm of the stethoscope with the alcohol wipe. Clean and store the sphygmomanometer, according to facility policy.

—— —— —— 26. Remove additional PPE, if used. Perform hand hygiene.

Skills Checklist to Accompany Fundamentals of Nursing:
The Art and Science of Person-Centered Care, 9th edition

Name _____ Date _____

Unit _____ Position _____

Instructor/Evaluator: _____ Position _____

Excellent	Satisfactory	Needs Practice	SKILL 26-1 **Using a Portable Bed Scale**	Comments
			Goal: The patient's weight is assessed accurately, without injury, and the patient experiences minimal discomfort.	
___	___	___	1. Check the medical order or nursing care plan for frequency of weight measurement. More frequent measurement of the patient's weight may be appropriate based on nursing judgment. Obtain the assistance of a second caregiver, based on the patient's mobility and ability to cooperate with the procedure.	
___	___	___	2. Perform hand hygiene and put on PPE, if indicated.	
___	___	___	3. Identify the patient.	
___	___	___	4. Close the curtains around the bed and close the door to the room if possible. Discuss the procedure with the patient and assess the patient's ability to assist with the procedure.	
___	___	___	5. Place a cover over the sling of the bed scale.	
___	___	___	6. Attach the sling to the bed scale. Lay the sheet or bath blanket in the sling. Turn on the scale. *Balance the scale so that weight reads 0.0.*	
___	___	___	7. Adjust the bed to a comfortable working position, usually elbow height of the caregiver (VHACEOSH, 2016). Position one caregiver on each side of the bed, if two caregivers are present. Raise side rail on the opposite side of the bed from where the scale is located, if not already in place. Cover the patient with the sheet or bath blanket. Remove other covers and any pillows.	
___	___	___	8. Turn the patient onto his or her side facing the side rail, keeping his or her body covered with the sheet or blanket. Remove the sling from the scale. Place the cover on the sling. Roll cover and sling lengthwise. Place rolled sling under the patient, making sure the patient is centered in the sling.	
___	___	___	9. Roll the patient back over the sling and onto the other side. Pull the sling through, as if placing sheet under patient, unrolling the sling as it is pulled through.	

Excellent	Satisfactory	Needs Practice	SKILL 26-1 **Using a Portable Bed Scale** *(Continued)*	Comments
—	—	—	10. Roll the scale over the bed so that the arms of the scale are directly over the patient. *Spread the base of the scale.* Lower the arms of the scale and place the arm hooks into the holes on the sling.	
—	—	—	11. Once the scale arms are hooked onto the sling, gradually elevate the sling so that the patient is lifted up off the bed. *Assess all tubes and drains, making sure that none have tension placed on them as the scale is lifted. Once the sling is no longer touching the bed, ensure that nothing else is hanging onto the sling (e.g., ventilator or IV tubing). If any tubing is connected to the patient, raise it up so that it is not adding any weight to the patient.*	
—	—	—	12. Note the weight reading on the scale. Slowly and gently, lower the patient back onto the bed. Disconnect the scale arms from the sling. Close the base of the scale and pull it away from the bed.	
—	—	—	13. Raise the side rail. Turn the patient to the side rail. Roll the sling up against the patient's backside.	
—	—	—	14. Raise the other side rail. Roll the patient back over the sling and up facing the other side rail. Remove the sling from the bed. Remove gloves, if used. Raise the remaining side rail.	
—	—	—	15. Cover the patient and help him or her to a position of comfort. Place the bed in the lowest position.	
—	—	—	16. Remove the disposable cover from the sling and discard in the appropriate receptacle.	
—	—	—	17. Remove additional PPE, if used. Clean equipment based on facility policy. Perform hand hygiene.	
—	—	—	18. Replace the scale and sling in the appropriate spot. Plug the scale into the electrical outlet.	

Skills Checklist to Accompany Fundamentals of Nursing:
The Art and Science of Person-Centered Care, 9th edition

Name _____   Date _____

Unit _____   Position _____

Instructor/Evaluator: _____   Position _____

Excellent	Satisfactory	Needs Practice	SKILL 26-2 ## Assessing the Neurologic, Musculoskeletal, and Peripheral Vascular Systems	Comments
			Goal: The assessments are completed without causing the patient to experience anxiety or discomfort, the findings are documented, and the appropriate referral is made to other health care professionals, as needed, for further evaluation.	
___	___	___	1. Perform hand hygiene and put on PPE, if indicated.	
___	___	___	2. Identify the patient.	
___	___	___	3. Close the curtains around the bed and close the door to the room, if possible. Explain the purpose of the neurologic, musculoskeletal, and peripheral vascular examinations and what you are going to do. Answer any questions.	
___	___	___	4. Help the patient undress, if needed, and provide a patient gown. Assist the patient to a supine position, if possible. Use the bath blanket to cover any exposed area other than the one being assessed.	
___	___	___	5. Begin with a survey of the patient's overall hygiene and physical appearance.	
___	___	___	6. Assess the patient's mental status.	
___	___	___	a. Evaluate level of consciousness.	
___	___	___	b. Evaluate the patient's orientation to person, place, and time.	
___	___	___	c. Assess memory (immediate recall and past memory).	
___	___	___	d. Evaluate the patient's ability to understand spoken and written word.	
___	___	___	7. Test cranial nerve (CN) function, as indicated.	
___	___	___	a. Ask the patient to close the eyes, occlude one nostril, and then identify the smell of different substances, such as coffee, chocolate, or alcohol. Repeat with other nostril.	
___	___	___	b. Test visual acuity and pupillary constriction.	
___	___	___	c. Move the patient's eyes through the six cardinal positions of gaze.	
___	___	___	d. Ask the patient to smile, frown, wrinkle the forehead, and puff out cheeks.	
___	___	___	e. Ask the patient to protrude tongue and push against the cheek with the tongue.	

Assessing the Neurologic, Musculoskeletal, and Peripheral Vascular Systems *(Continued)*

Excellent	Satisfactory	Needs Practice		Comments
——	——	——	f. Palpate the jaw muscles. Ask the patient to open and clench jaws. Stroke the patient's face with a cotton ball.	
——	——	——	g. Test hearing with the whispered voice test.	
——	——	——	h. Put on gloves. Ask patient to open mouth. While observing soft palate, ask patient to say "ah"; observe upward movement of the soft palate. Test the gag reflex by touching the posterior pharynx with the tongue depressor. Explain to patient that this may be uncomfortable. Ask the patient to swallow. Remove gloves.	
——	——	——	i. Place your hands on the patient's shoulders while he or she shrugs against resistance. Then place your hand on the patient's left cheek, then the right cheek, and have the patient push against it.	
——	——	——	8. Check the patient's ability to move his or her neck. Ask the patient to touch his or her chin to the chest and to each shoulder, then move each ear to the corresponding shoulder, and then tip the head back as far as possible.	
——	——	——	9. Inspect the upper extremities. Observe for skin color, presence of lesions, rashes, and muscle mass. Palpate for skin temperature, texture, and presence of masses.	
——	——	——	10. Ask the patient to extend arms forward and then rapidly turn palms up and down.	
——	——	——	11. Ask the patient to flex upper arm and to resist examiner's opposing force.	
——	——	——	12. Inspect and palpate the hands, fingers, wrists, and elbow joints.	
——	——	——	13. Ask the patient to bend and straighten the elbow, and flex and extend the wrists and hands.	
——	——	——	14. Palpate the skin and the radial and brachial pulses. Assess the pulse rate, quality or amplitude, and rhythm. Test capillary refill.	
——	——	——	15. Have the patient squeeze your index and middle fingers.	
——	——	——	16. Assist the patient to a supine position. Palpate and then use the bell of the stethoscope to auscultate the femoral pulses in the groin, if not done during assessment of the abdomen. Note the strength of the pulse and grade it as with peripheral pulses.	
——	——	——	17. Examine the lower extremities. Inspect the legs and feet for color, lesions, varicosities, hair growth, nail growth, edema, and muscle mass.	

SKILL 26-2

Assessing the Neurologic, Musculoskeletal, and Peripheral Vascular Systems *(Continued)*

Excellent	Satisfactory	Needs Practice		Comments
——	——	——	18. Assess for pitting edema in the lower extremities by pressing fingers into the skin at the pretibial area and dorsum of the foot. If an indentation remains in the skin after the fingers have been lifted, pitting edema is present.	
——	——	——	19. Palpate for pulses and skin temperature at the posterior tibial, dorsalis pedis, and popliteal areas. Assess the pulse rate, quality or amplitude, and rhythm. Test capillary refill.	
——	——	——	20. Ask the patient to move one leg laterally with the knee straight to test abduction of the hip. Keeping knee straight, move leg medially to test adduction of the hip. Repeat with other leg.	
——	——	——	21. Ask the patient to raise the thigh against the resistance of your hand; next have the patient push outward against the resistance of your hand; then have the patient pull backward against the resistance of your hand. Repeat on the opposite side.	
——	——	——	22. Ask the patient to dorsiflex and then plantarflex both feet against opposing resistance.	
——	——	——	23. As needed, assist the patient to a standing position. Observe the patient as he or she walks with a regular gait, on the toes, on the heels, and then heel to toe.	
——	——	——	24. Perform the Romberg's test; ask the patient to stand straight with feet together, both eyes closed with arms at side. Wait 20 seconds and observe for patient swaying and ability to maintain balance. Be alert to prevent patient fall or injury related to losing balance during this assessment.	
——	——	——	25. Assist the patient to a comfortable position.	
——	——	——	26. Remove PPE, if used. Perform hand hygiene. Continue with assessments of specific body systems, as appropriate, or indicated. Initiate appropriate referral to other health care providers for further evaluation, as indicated.	

Skills Checklist to Accompany Fundamentals of Nursing:
The Art and Science of Person-Centered Care, 9th edition

Name _____ Date _____

Unit _____ Position _____

Instructor/Evaluator: _____ Position _____

SKILL 27-1

Performing a Situational Assessment

Goal: The patient's situation (including airway, breathing, and circulation; level of consciousness, orientation, and speech; and environment) is assessed accurately without injury, and the patient experiences only minimal discomfort.

Excellent	Satisfactory	Needs Practice		Comments
——	——	——	1. Perform hand hygiene and put on PPE, if indicated.	
——	——	——	2. Identify the patient. Explain the purpose of the assessment to the patient.	
——	——	——	3. Assess for data that suggest a problem with the patient's airway, breathing, or circulation. If a problem is present, identify if it is urgent or nonurgent in nature.	
——	——	——	4. Assess the patient's level of consciousness, orientation, and speech. Observe the patient's behavior and affect.	
——	——	——	5. Assess the patency of an oxygen delivery device, if in use.	
——	——	——	6. Survey the patient's environment. Assess the bed position and call bell location. Bed should be in the lowest position and the call bell (based on specific patient care setting) should be within the patient's reach.	
——	——	——	7. Assess for clutter and hazards. Remove excess equipment, supplies, furniture, and other objects from rooms and walkways. Pay particular attention to high traffic areas and the route to the bathroom.	
——	——	——	8. Note the presence and location of appropriate emergency equipment, based on individual patient situation.	
——	——	——	9. Note the presence and location of appropriate assistive devices and mobility aids, based on individual patient situation. Ensure any devices are within the patient's reach.	
——	——	——	10. Assess for the presence of an intravenous access and/or infusion. Assess patency of the device and the insertion site. If an infusion is present, assess the solution and rate.	
——	——	——	11. Assess for the presence of any tubes, such as gastric tubes, chest tubes, surgical drains, or urinary catheters. Assess patency of device and insertion site.	
——	——	——	12. Provide a bedside commode and/or urinal/bedpan, if appropriate. Ensure that it is near the bed at all times.	
——	——	——	13. Ensure that the bedside table, telephone, and other personal items are within the patient's reach at all times.	

Excellent	Satisfactory	Needs Practice	SKILL 27-1 **Performing a Situational Assessment** *(Continued)*
			Comments
――	――	――	14. Consider what further assessments should be completed and additional interventions that may be indicated. Identify problems that need to be reported and whom to contact.
――	――	――	15. Remove PPE, if used. Perform hand hygiene.

Skills Checklist to Accompany Fundamentals of Nursing:
The Art and Science of Person-Centered Care, 9th edition

Name _____ Date _____

Unit _____ Position _____

Instructor/Evaluator: _____ Position _____

Excellent	Satisfactory	Needs Practice	SKILL 27-2 **Applying an Extremity Restraint**	Comments
			Goal: The patient is constrained by the restraint, remains free from injury, and the restraint does not interfere with therapeutic devices.	
——	——	——	1. Determine the need for restraints. Assess the patient's physical condition, behavior, and mental status.	
——	——	——	2. Confirm facility policy for the application of restraints. *Secure an order from the primary care provider, or validate that the order has been obtained within the required time frame.*	
——	——	——	3. Perform hand hygiene and put on PPE, if indicated.	
——	——	——	4. Identify the patient.	
——	——	——	5. Explain the reason for restraint use to patient and family. Clarify how care will be given and how needs will be met. Explain that restraint is a temporary measure.	
——	——	——	6. Include the patient's family and/or significant others in the plan of care.	
——	——	——	7. Apply restraint according to the manufacturer's directions:	
——	——	——	a. Choose the least restrictive type of device that allows the greatest possible degree of mobility.	
——	——	——	b. Pad bony prominences.	
——	——	——	c. Wrap the restraint around the extremity with the soft part in contact with the skin. If a hand mitt is being used, pull over the hand with cushion to the palmar aspect of the hand.	
——	——	——	8. Secure in place with the Velcro straps or other mechanism, depending on specific restraint device. Depending on the characteristics of the specific restraint, it may be necessary to tie a knot in the restraint ties, to ensure the restraint remains secure on the extremity.	
——	——	——	9. *Ensure that two fingers can be inserted between the restraint and patient's extremity.*	
——	——	——	10. Maintain restrained extremity in normal anatomic position. *Use a quick-release knot to tie the restraint to the bed frame, not side rail.* The restraint may also be attached to a chair frame. The site should not be readily accessible to the patient.	
——	——	——	11. Remove PPE, if used. Perform hand hygiene.	

Applying an Extremity Restraint *(Continued)*

Excellent	Satisfactory	Needs Practice		Comments
——	——	——	12. Assess the patient at least every hour or according to facility policy. Assessment should include the placement of the restraint, neurovascular assessment of the affected extremity, and skin integrity. In addition, assess for signs of sensory deprivation, such as increased sleeping, daydreaming, anxiety, panic, and hallucinations. Monitor the patient's vital signs.	
——	——	——	13. ***Remove the restraint at least every 2 hours, or according to facility policy and patient need.*** Perform range-of-motion (ROM) exercises.	
——	——	——	14. Evaluate the patient for continued need of restraint. Reapply restraint only if continued need is evident and order is still valid.	
——	——	——	15. Reassure the patient at regular intervals. Provide continued explanation of rationale for interventions, reorientation if necessary, and plan of care. ***Keep the call bell within the patient's easy reach.***	

Skills Checklist to Accompany Fundamentals of Nursing:
The Art and Science of Person-Centered Care, 9th edition

Name _____ Date _____

Unit _____ Position _____

Instructor/Evaluator: _____ Position _____

Excellent	Satisfactory	Needs Practice	SKILL 29-1 **Administering Oral Medications**	Comments
			Goal: The patient swallows the prescribed medication at the proper time.	
⎯⎯	⎯⎯	⎯⎯	1. Gather equipment. Check each medication order against the original in the medical record, according to facility policy. Clarify any inconsistencies. Check the patient's medical record for allergies.	
⎯⎯	⎯⎯	⎯⎯	2. Know the actions, special nursing considerations, safe dose ranges, purpose of administration, and potential adverse effects of the medications to be administered. Consider the appropriateness of the medication for this patient.	
⎯⎯	⎯⎯	⎯⎯	3. Perform hand hygiene.	
⎯⎯	⎯⎯	⎯⎯	4. Move the medication supply system to the outside of the patient's room or prepare for administration at the medication supply system in the medication area. Alternatively, access the medication administration supply system at or inside the patient's room.	
⎯⎯	⎯⎯	⎯⎯	5. Unlock the medication supply system or drawer. Enter pass code into the computer and scan employee identification, if required.	
⎯⎯	⎯⎯	⎯⎯	6. *Prepare medications for one patient at a time.*	
⎯⎯	⎯⎯	⎯⎯	7. Read the eMAR/MAR and select the proper medication from the medication supply system or patient's medication drawer.	
⎯⎯	⎯⎯	⎯⎯	8. Compare the medication label with the eMAR/MAR. Check expiration dates and perform calculations, if necessary. Scan the bar code on the package, if required.	
⎯⎯	⎯⎯	⎯⎯	9. Prepare the required medications:	
⎯⎯	⎯⎯	⎯⎯	a. *Unit dose packages:* **Do not open the wrapper until at the bedside.** Keep opioids and medications that require special nursing assessments separate from other medication packages.	
⎯⎯	⎯⎯	⎯⎯	b. *Multidose containers:* When removing tablets or capsules from a multidose bottle, pour the necessary number into the bottle cap and then place the tablets or capsules in a medication cup. Break only scored tablets, if necessary, to obtain the proper dosage. Do not touch tablets or capsules with hands.	

Excellent	Satisfactory	Needs Practice		Comments

Administering Oral Medications *(Continued)*

Excellent	Satisfactory	Needs Practice		Comments
——	——	——	c. *Liquid medication in multidose bottle:* When pouring liquid medications out of a multidose bottle, hold the bottle so the label is against the palm. Use the appropriate measuring device when pouring liquids, and read the amount of medication at the bottom of the meniscus at eye level. Wipe the lip of the bottle with a paper towel.	
——	——	——	10. *Depending on facility policy, the third check of the label may occur at this point. If so, when all medications for one patient have been prepared, recheck the labels with the eMAR/MAR before taking the medications to the patient. However, many facilities require the third check to occur at the bedside, after identifying the patient.*	
——	——	——	11. Replace any multidose containers in the patient's drawer or medication supply system. *Lock the medication supply system before leaving it.*	
——	——	——	12. Transport medications to the patient's bedside carefully, and keep the medications in sight at all times.	
——	——	——	13. *Ensure that the patient receives the medications at the correct time.*	
——	——	——	14. Perform hand hygiene and put on PPE, if indicated.	
——	——	——	15. *Identify the patient. Compare the information with the eMAR/MAR. The patient should be identified using at least two of the following methods* (The Joint Commission, 2018):	
——	——	——	a. Check the name on the patient's identification band.	
——	——	——	b. Check the identification number on the patient's identification band.	
——	——	——	c. Check the birth date on the patient's identification band.	
——	——	——	d. Ask the patient to state his or her name and birth date, based on facility policy.	
——	——	——	16. *Complete necessary assessments before administering medications. Check the patient's allergy bracelet or ask the patient about allergies. Explain the purpose and action of each medication to the patient.*	
——	——	——	17. Scan the patient's bar code on the identification band, if required.	
——	——	——	18. *Based on facility policy, the third check of the medication label may occur at this point. If so, recheck the label with the eMAR/MAR before administering the medications to the patient.*	

Administering Oral Medications *(Continued)*

Excellent	Satisfactory	Needs Practice		Comments
——	——	——	19. Assist the patient to an upright or lateral (side-lying) position.	
——	——	——	20. Administer medications:	
——	——	——	a. Offer water or other permitted fluids with pills, capsules, tablets, and some liquid medications.	
——	——	——	b. Ask whether the patient prefers to take the medications by hand or in a cup.	
——	——	——	21. ***Remain with the patient until each medication is swallowed. Never leave medication at the patient's bedside.***	
——	——	——	22. Assist the patient to a comfortable position. Remove PPE, if used. Perform hand hygiene.	
——	——	——	23. Document the administration of the medication immediately after administration.	
——	——	——	24. Evaluate the patient's response to the medication within the appropriate time frame.	

Skills Checklist to Accompany Fundamentals of Nursing:
The Art and Science of Person-Centered Care, 9th edition

Name _____ Date _____

Unit _____ Position _____

Instructor/Evaluator: _____ Position _____

Excellent	Satisfactory	Needs Practice	SKILL 29-2 **Removing Medication From an Ampule**	Comments
			Goal: The proper dose of medication is removed in a sterile manner, and is free from glass shards.	
____	____	____	1. Gather equipment. Check the medication order against the original order in the medical record, according to facility policy. Clarify any inconsistencies. Check the patient's health record for allergies.	
____	____	____	2. Know the actions, special nursing considerations, safe dose ranges, purpose of administration, and adverse effects of the medications to be administered. Consider the appropriateness of the medication for this patient.	
____	____	____	3. Perform hand hygiene.	
____	____	____	4. Move the medication supply system to the outside of the patient's room or prepare for administration at the medication supply system in the medication area. Alternatively, access the medication administration supply system at or inside the patient's room.	
____	____	____	5. Unlock the medication supply system or drawer. Enter pass code and scan employee identification, if required.	
____	____	____	6. *Prepare medications for one patient at a time.*	
____	____	____	7. Read the eMAR/MAR and select the proper medication from the medication supply system or the patient's medication drawer.	
____	____	____	8. Compare the label with the eMAR/MAR. Check expiration dates and perform calculations, if necessary. Scan the bar code on the package, if required.	
____	____	____	9. Tap the stem of the ampule or twist your wrist quickly while holding the ampule vertically.	
____	____	____	10. Using the antimicrobial swab, scrub the neck of the ampule (Dolan et al., 2016). Wrap a small sterile gauze pad around the neck of the ampule.	
____	____	____	11. Breaking away from your body, use a snapping motion to break off the top of the ampule along the scored line at its neck. *Always break away from your body.*	
____	____	____	12. Attach filter needle to syringe. Remove the cap from the filter needle by pulling it straight off.	

Removing Medication From an Ampule *(Continued)*

Excellent	Satisfactory	Needs Practice		Comments

Excellent	Satisfactory	Needs Practice		
——	——	——	13. Withdraw medication in the amount ordered plus a small amount more (approximately 30% more). *Do not inject air into the solution. While inserting the filter needle into the ampule, be careful not to touch the rim.* Use either of the following methods to withdraw the medication:	
——	——	——	a. Insert the tip of the needle into the ampule, which is upright on a flat surface, and withdraw fluid into the syringe. *Touch the plunger only at the knob.*	
——	——	——	b. Insert the tip of the needle into the ampule and invert the ampule. Keep the needle centered and not touching the sides of the ampule. Withdraw fluid into syringe. *Touch the plunger only at the knob.*	
——	——	——	14. Wait until the needle has been withdrawn to tap the syringe and expel the air carefully by pushing on the plunger. *Check the amount of medication in the syringe with the medication dose and discard any surplus, according to facility policy.*	
——	——	——	15. *Depending on facility policy, the third check of the label may occur at this point. If so, when all medications for one patient have been prepared, recheck the labels with the eMAR/MAR before taking the medications to the patient. However, many facilities require the third check to occur at the bedside, after identifying the patient.*	
——	——	——	16. *Engage safety guard on filter needle and remove the needle. Discard the filter needle in a suitable container. Attach appropriate administration device to syringe.*	
——	——	——	17. Discard the ampule in a suitable container.	
——	——	——	18. *Lock the medication supply system before leaving it.*	
——	——	——	19. Perform hand hygiene.	
——	——	——	20. Proceed with administration, based on prescribed route.	

Skills Checklist to Accompany Fundamentals of Nursing:
The Art and Science of Person-Centered Care, 9th edition

Name _____   Date _____

Unit _____   Position _____

Instructor/Evaluator: _____   Position _____

Excellent	Satisfactory	Needs Practice	SKILL 29-3 **Removing Medication From a Vial**	Comments
			Goal: The proper dosage of medication is withdrawn into a syringe using sterile technique.	
____	____	____	1. Gather equipment. Check the medication order against the original order in the medical record, according to facility policy. Clarify any inconsistencies. Check the patient's health record for allergies.	
____	____	____	2. Know the actions, special nursing considerations, safe dose ranges, purpose of administration, and adverse effects of the medications to be administered. Consider the appropriateness of the medication for this patient.	
____	____	____	3. Perform hand hygiene.	
____	____	____	4. Move the medication supply system to the outside of the patient's room or prepare for administration at the medication supply system in the medication area. Alternatively, access the medication administration supply system at or inside the patient's room.	
____	____	____	5. Unlock the medication supply system or drawer. Enter pass code and scan employee identification, if required.	
____	____	____	6. *Prepare medications for one patient at a time.*	
____	____	____	7. Read the eMAR/MAR and select the proper medication from the medication supply system or the patient's medication drawer.	
____	____	____	8. Compare the label with the eMAR/MAR. Check expiration dates and perform calculations, if necessary. Scan the bar code on the package, if required.	
____	____	____	9. Remove the metal or plastic cap on the vial that protects the self-sealing stopper.	
____	____	____	10. *Scrub the self-sealing stopper top with the antimicrobial swab and allow to dry.*	
____	____	____	11. Remove the cap from the needle or blunt cannula by pulling it straight off. If the vial in use is a multidose vial, touch the plunger only at the knob and draw back an amount of air into the syringe that is equal to the specific dose of medication to be withdrawn. If the vial in use is a single-use vial, there is no need to draw air into the syringe.	

Excellent	Satisfactory	Needs Practice	SKILL 29-3 **Removing Medication From a Vial** *(Continued)*	Comments
—	—	—	12. Hold the vial on a flat surface. Pierce the self-sealing stopper in the center with the needle tip and inject the measured air into the space above the solution. *Do not inject air into the solution.* If the vial in use is a single-use vial, there is no need to inject air into the vial.	
—	—	—	13. Invert the vial. *Keep the tip of the needle or blunt cannula below the fluid level.*	
—	—	—	14. Hold the vial in one hand and use the other to withdraw the medication. *Touch the plunger only at the knob. Draw up the prescribed amount of medication while holding the syringe vertically and at eye level.*	
—	—	—	15. If any air bubbles accumulate in the syringe, tap the barrel of the syringe sharply and move the needle past the fluid into the air space to re-inject the air bubble into the vial. Return the needle tip to the solution and continue withdrawal of the medication.	
—	—	—	16. After the correct dose is withdrawn, remove the needle from the vial and carefully replace the cap over the needle. Some facilities require changing the needle, if one was used to withdraw the medication, before administering the medication.	
—	—	—	17. *Check the amount of medication in the syringe with the medication dose and discard any surplus.*	
—	—	—	18. *Depending on facility policy, the third check of the label may occur at this point. If so, when all medications for one patient have been prepared, recheck the labels with the eMAR/MAR before taking the medications to the patient. However, many facilities require the third check to occur at the bedside, after identifying the patient.*	
—	—	—	19. *If a multidose vial is being used, label the vial with the date and time opened and the beyond-use date (see Special Considerations), and store the vial containing the remaining medication according to facility policy.* Limit the use of multiple-dose vials and dedicate them to a single patient whenever possible (CDC, n.d.b).	
—	—	—	20. *Lock the medication supply system before leaving it.*	
—	—	—	21. Perform hand hygiene.	
—	—	—	22. Proceed with administration, based on prescribed route.	

Skills Checklist to Accompany Fundamentals of Nursing:
The Art and Science of Person-Centered Care, 9th edition

Name _____ Date _____

Unit _____ Position _____

Instructor/Evaluator: _____ Position _____

Excellent	Satisfactory	Needs Practice	SKILL 29-4 **Mixing Medications From Two Vials in One Syringe**	Comments
			Goal: The proper dosage of medication is withdrawn into a syringe using sterile technique.	
___	___	___	1. Gather equipment. Check medication order against the original order in the medical record, according to facility policy.	
___	___	___	2. Know the actions, special nursing considerations, safe dose ranges, purpose of administration, and adverse effects of the medications to be administered. Consider the appropriateness of the medication for this patient.	
___	___	___	3. Perform hand hygiene.	
___	___	___	4. Move the medication supply system to the outside of the patient's room or prepare for administration at the medication supply system in the medication area. Alternatively, access the medication administration supply system at or inside the patient's room.	
___	___	___	5. Unlock the medication supply system or drawer. Enter pass code and scan employee identification, if required.	
___	___	___	6. *Prepare medications for one patient at a time.*	
___	___	___	7. Read the eMAR/MAR and select the proper medications from the medication supply system or the patient's medication drawer.	
___	___	___	8. Compare the labels with the eMAR/MAR. Check expiration dates and perform dosage calculations, if necessary. Scan the bar code on the package, if required.	
___	___	___	9. If necessary, remove the cap that protects the self-sealing stopper on each vial.	
___	___	___	10. *If medication is a suspension (e.g., a modified insulin, such as NPH insulin), roll and agitate the vial to mix it well.*	
___	___	___	11. *Scrub the self-sealing stopper top with the antimicrobial swab and allow to dry.*	
___	___	___	12. Remove cap from needle by pulling it straight off. Touch the plunger only at the knob. Draw back an amount of air into the syringe that is equal to the dose of modified insulin to be withdrawn.	

Mixing Medications From Two Vials in One Syringe (Continued)

Excellent	Satisfactory	Needs Practice		Comments
——	——	——	13. Hold the modified vial on a flat surface. Pierce the self-sealing stopper in the center with the needle tip and inject the measured air into the space above the solution. Do not inject air into the solution. Withdraw the needle.	
——	——	——	14. Draw back an amount of air into the syringe that is equal to the dose of unmodified insulin to be withdrawn.	
——	——	——	15. Hold the unmodified vial on a flat surface. Pierce the self-sealing stopper in the center with the needle tip and inject the measured air into the space above the solution. Do not inject air into the solution. Keep the needle in the vial.	
——	——	——	16. Invert the vial of unmodified insulin. Hold the vial in one hand and use the other to withdraw the medication. *Touch the plunger only at the knob. Draw up the prescribed amount of medication while holding the syringe at eye level and vertically.* Turn the vial over and then remove the needle from the vial.	
——	——	——	17. Check that there are no air bubbles in the syringe.	
——	——	——	18. *Check the amount of medication in the syringe with the medication dose and discard any surplus.*	
——	——	——	19. *Recheck the vial label with the eMAR/MAR.*	
——	——	——	20. Calculate the endpoint on the syringe for the combined insulin amount by adding the number of units for each dose together.	
——	——	——	21. Insert the needle into the modified vial and invert it, taking care not to push the plunger and inject medication from the syringe into the vial. Invert vial of modified insulin. Hold the vial in one hand and use the other to withdraw the medication. *Touch the plunger only at the knob. Draw up the prescribed amount of medication while holding the syringe at eye level and vertically. Take care to withdraw only the prescribed amount.* Turn the vial over and then remove the needle from the vial. Carefully recap the needle. Carefully replace the cap over the needle.	
——	——	——	22. *Check the amount of medication in the syringe with the medication dose.*	
——	——	——	23. *Depending on facility policy, the third check of the label may occur at this point. If so, recheck the label with the MAR before taking the medications to the patient. However, many facilities require the third check to occur at the bedside, after identifying the patient.*	

Mixing Medications From Two Vials in
One Syrinage *(Continued)*

Excellent	Satisfactory	Needs Practice		Comments
—	—	—	24. *Label the vials with the date and time opened and beyond-use date, and store the vials containing the remaining medication, according to facility policy.*	
—	—	—	25. *Lock the medication supply system before leaving it.*	
—	—	—	26. Perform hand hygiene.	
—	—	—	27. Proceed with administration, based on prescribed route.	

36

Name _____ Date _____

Unit _____ Position _____

Instructor/Evaluator: _____ Position _____

SKILL 29-5

Administering an Intradermal Injection

Goal: Medication is safely injected intradermally, causing a wheal to appear at the site of the injection.

Excellent	Satisfactory	Needs Practice		Comments
—	—	—	1. Gather equipment. Check each medication order against the original order in the medical record according to facility policy. Clarify any inconsistencies. Check the patient's health record for allergies.	
—	—	—	2. Know the actions, special nursing considerations, safe dose ranges, purpose of administration, and adverse effects of the medications to be administered. Consider the appropriateness of the medication for this patient.	
—	—	—	3. Perform hand hygiene.	
—	—	—	4. Move the medication supply system to the outside of the patient's room or prepare for administration at the medication supply system in the medication area. Alternatively, access the medication administration supply system at or inside the patient's room.	
—	—	—	5. Unlock the medication supply system or drawer. Enter pass code and scan employee identification, if required.	
—	—	—	6. *Prepare medications for one patient at a time.*	
—	—	—	7. Read the eMAR/MAR and select the proper medication from the medication supply system or the patient's medication drawer.	
—	—	—	8. Compare the label with the eMAR/MAR. Check expiration dates and perform calculations, if necessary. Scan the bar code on the package, if required.	
—	—	—	9. If necessary, withdraw the medication from an ampule or vial.	
—	—	—	10. *Depending on facility policy, the third check of the label may occur at this point. If so, when all medications for one patient have been prepared, recheck the labels with the eMAR/MAR before taking the medications to the patient. However, many facilities require the third check to occur at the bedside, after identifying the patient.*	
—	—	—	11. *Lock the medication supply system before leaving it.*	
—	—	—	12. Transport medications to the patient's bedside carefully, and keep the medications in sight at all times.	

SKILL 29-5

Administering an Intradermal
Injection *(Continued)*

Excellent	Satisfactory	Needs Practice		Comments

Excellent	Satisfactory	Needs Practice	
——	——	——	13. *Ensure that the patient receives the medications at the correct time.*
——	——	——	14. Perform hand hygiene and put on PPE, if indicated.
——	——	——	15. *Identify the patient. Compare the information with the eMAR/MAR. The patient should be identified using at least two of the following methods* (The Joint Commission, 2018):
——	——	——	a. Check the name on the patient's identification band.
——	——	——	b. Check the identification number on the patient's identification band.
——	——	——	c. Check the birth date on the patient's identification band.
——	——	——	d. Ask the patient to state his or her name and birth date, based on facility policy.
——	——	——	16. Close the door to the room or pull the bedside curtain.
——	——	——	17. *Complete necessary assessments before administering medications. Check allergy bracelet or ask the patient about allergies. Explain the purpose and action of the medication to the patient.*
——	——	——	18. Scan the patient's bar code on the identification band, if required.
——	——	——	19. *Based on facility policy, the third check of the label may occur at this point. If so, recheck the labels with the eMAR/MAR before administering the medications to the patient.*
——	——	——	20. Put on clean gloves.
——	——	——	21. Select an appropriate administration site. Assist the patient to the appropriate position for the site chosen. Drape, as needed, to expose only site area to be used.
——	——	——	22. Cleanse the site with an antimicrobial swab while wiping with a firm, circular motion and moving outward from the injection site. Allow the skin to dry.
——	——	——	23. Remove the needle cap with the nondominant hand by pulling it straight off.
——	——	——	24. Use the nondominant hand to spread the skin taut over the injection site.
——	——	——	25. Hold the syringe in the dominant hand, between the thumb and forefinger with the bevel of the needle up.

Excellent	Satisfactory	Needs Practice	

SKILL 29-5

Administering an Intradermal Injection *(Continued)*

Comments

Excellent	Satisfactory	Needs Practice		
——	——	——	26. Hold the syringe at a 5- to 15-degree angle from the site. Place the needle almost flat against the patient's skin, bevel side up, and insert the needle into the skin. Insert the needle only about ⅛ in with entire bevel under the skin.	
——	——	——	27. Once the needle is in place, steady the lower end of the syringe. Slide your dominant hand to the end of the plunger.	
——	——	——	28. Slowly inject the agent while watching for a small wheal to appear.	
——	——	——	29. Withdraw the needle quickly at the same angle that it was inserted. Do not recap the used needle. Engage the safety shield or needle guard.	
——	——	——	30. *Do not massage the area after removing needle. Tell the patient not to rub or scratch the site. If necessary, gently blot the site with a dry gauze square. Do not apply pressure or rub the site.*	
——	——	——	31. Assist the patient to a position of comfort.	
——	——	——	32. Discard the needle and syringe in the appropriate receptacle.	
——	——	——	33. Remove gloves and additional PPE, if used. Perform hand hygiene.	
——	——	——	34. Document the administration of the medication immediately after administration.	
——	——	——	35. Evaluate the patient's response to the medication within the appropriate time frame.	
——	——	——	36. Observe the area for signs of a reaction at determined intervals after administration. Inform the patient of the need for inspection.	

Skills Checklist to Accompany Fundamentals of Nursing:
The Art and Science of Person-Centered Care, 9th edition

Name _____   Date _____

Unit _____   Position _____

Instructor/Evaluator: _____   Position _____

Excellent	Satisfactory	Needs Practice	SKILL 29-6 **Administering a Subcutaneous Injection** **Goal**: The patient safely receives medication via the subcutaneous route.	Comments
___	___	___	1. Gather equipment. Check each medication order against the original order in the medical record, according to facility policy. Clarify any inconsistencies. Check the patient's health record for allergies.	
___	___	___	2. Know the actions, special nursing considerations, safe dose ranges, purpose of administration, and adverse effects of the medications to be administered. Consider the appropriateness of the medication for this patient.	
___	___	___	3. Perform hand hygiene.	
___	___	___	4. Move the medication supply system to the outside of the patient's room or prepare for administration at the medication supply system in the medication area. Alternatively, access the medication administration supply system at or inside the patient's room.	
___	___	___	5. Unlock the medication supply system or drawer. Enter pass code and scan employee identification, if required.	
___	___	___	6. *Prepare medications for one patient at a time.*	
___	___	___	7. Read the eMAR/MAR and select the proper medication from the medication supply system or the patient's medication drawer.	
___	___	___	8. Compare the medication label with the eMAR/MAR. Check expiration dates and perform calculations, if necessary. Scan the bar code on the package, if required.	
___	___	___	9. If necessary, withdraw medication from an ampule or vial.	
___	___	___	10. *Depending on facility policy, the third check of the label may occur at this point. If so, when all medications for one patient have been prepared, recheck the labels with the eMAR/MAR before taking the medications to the patient. However, many facilities require the third check to occur at the bedside, after identifying the patient.*	
___	___	___	11. *Lock the medication supply system before leaving it.*	
___	___	___	12. Transport medications to the patient's bedside carefully, and keep the medications in sight at all times.	

SKILL 29-6

Administering a Subcutaneous Injection *(Continued)*

Excellent	Satisfactory	Needs Practice		Comments
——	——	——	13. *Ensure that the patient receives the medications at the correct time.*	
——	——	——	14. Perform hand hygiene and put on PPE, if indicated.	
——	——	——	15. *Identify the patient. Compare the information with the eMAR/MAR. The patient should be identified using at least two of the following methods* (The Joint Commission, 2018):	
——	——	——	a. Check the name on the patient's identification band.	
——	——	——	b. Check the identification number on the patient's identification band.	
——	——	——	c. Check the birth date on the patient's identification band.	
——	——	——	d. Ask the patient to state his or her name and birth date, based on facility policy.	
——	——	——	16. Close the door to the room or pull the bedside curtain.	
——	——	——	17. *Complete necessary assessments before administering medications. Check the patient's allergy bracelet or ask the patient about allergies.* Explain the purpose and action of the medication to the patient.	
——	——	——	18. Scan the patient's bar code on the identification band, if required.	
——	——	——	19. *Based on facility policy, the third check of the label may occur at this point. If so, recheck the labels with the eMAR/MAR before administering the medications to the patient.*	
——	——	——	20. Put on clean gloves.	
——	——	——	21. Select an appropriate administration site.	
——	——	——	22. Assist the patient to the appropriate position for the site chosen. Drape, as needed, to expose only site area to be used.	
——	——	——	23. Identify the appropriate landmarks for the site chosen.	
——	——	——	24. Cleanse the area around the injection site with an antimicrobial swab. Use a firm, circular motion while moving outward from the injection site. Allow the area to dry.	
——	——	——	25. Remove the needle cap with the nondominant hand, pulling it straight off.	
——	——	——	26. Create a skin fold, if necessary, by pinching the area surrounding the injection site. Alternatively, spread the skin taut at the site, based on assessment of the patient and needle length used for the injection.	

Administering a Subcutaneous Injection *(Continued)*

Excellent	Satisfactory	Needs Practice		Comments
___	___	___	27. Hold the syringe in the dominant hand between the thumb and forefinger. Inject the needle quickly at a 45- or 90-degree angle, depending on the amount of underlying subcutaneous tissue.	
___	___	___	28. If pinching is used, once the needle is inserted, release the skin and stabilize the base of the needle to avoid injecting into the compressed tissue. Slide your dominant hand to the end of the plunger. Avoid moving the syringe.	
___	___	___	29. Inject the medication slowly (at a rate of 10 sec/mL).	
___	___	___	30. Withdraw the needle quickly at the same angle at which it was inserted, while supporting the surrounding tissue with your nondominant hand.	
___	___	___	31. Do not recap the used needle. Engage the safety shield or needle guard.	
___	___	___	32. If blood or clear fluid appears at the site after withdrawing the needle, use a gauze square to apply gentle pressure to the site. ***Do not massage the site.***	
___	___	___	33. Assist the patient to a position of comfort.	
___	___	___	34. Discard the needle and syringe in the appropriate receptacle.	
___	___	___	35. Remove gloves and additional PPE, if used. Perform hand hygiene.	
___	___	___	36. Document the administration of the medication immediately after administration.	
___	___	___	37. Evaluate the patient's response to the medication within the appropriate time frame for the particular medication.	

Skills Checklist to Accompany Fundamentals of Nursing:
The Art and Science of Person-Centered Care, 9th edition

Name _____   Date _____

Unit _____   Position _____

Instructor/Evaluator: _____   Position _____

SKILL 29-7
Administering an Intramuscular Injection

Goal: The patient safely receives the medication via the intramuscular route using a Z-track method.

Excellent	Satisfactory	Needs Practice		Comments
___	___	___	1. Gather equipment. Check each medication order against the original order in the health record according to facility policy. Clarify any inconsistencies. Check the patient's health record for allergies.	
___	___	___	2. Know the actions, special nursing considerations, safe dose ranges, purpose of administration, and adverse effects of the medications to be administered. Consider the appropriateness of the medication for this patient.	
___	___	___	3. Perform hand hygiene.	
___	___	___	4. Move the medication supply system to the outside of the patient's room or prepare for administration at the medication supply system in the medication area. Alternatively, access the medication administration supply system at or inside the patient's room.	
___	___	___	5. Unlock the medication supply system or drawer. Enter pass code and scan employee identification, if required.	
___	___	___	6. *Prepare medications for one patient at a time.*	
___	___	___	7. Read the eMAR/MAR and select the proper medication from medication supply system or the patient's medication drawer.	
___	___	___	8. Compare the label with the eMAR/MAR. Check expiration dates and perform calculations, if necessary. Scan the bar code on the package, if required.	
___	___	___	9. If necessary, withdraw medication from an ampule or vial.	
___	___	___	10. *Depending on facility policy, the third check of the label may occur at this point. If so, when all medications for one patient have been prepared, recheck the labels with the eMAR/MAR before taking the medications to the patient. However, many facilities require the third check to occur at the bedside, after identifying the patient.*	
___	___	___	11. *Lock the medication supply system before leaving it.*	
___	___	___	12. Transport medications to the patient's bedside carefully, and keep the medications in sight at all times.	

Administering an Intramuscular Injection *(Continued)*

Excellent	Satisfactory	Needs Practice		Comments
——	——	——	13. *Ensure that the patient receives the medications at the correct time.*	
——	——	——	14. Perform hand hygiene and put on PPE, if indicated.	
——	——	——	15. *Identify the patient. Compare the information with the eMAR/MAR. The patient should be identified using at least two of the following methods* (The Joint Commission, 2018):	
——	——	——	a. Check the name on the patient's identification band.	
——	——	——	b. Check the identification number on the patient's identification band.	
——	——	——	c. Check the birth date on the patient's identification band.	
——	——	——	d. Ask the patient to state his or her name and birth date, based on facility policy.	
——	——	——	16. Close the door to the room or pull the bedside curtain.	
——	——	——	17. *Complete necessary assessments before administering medications. Check the patient's allergy bracelet or ask the patient about allergies. Explain the purpose and action of the medication to the patient.*	
——	——	——	18. Scan the patient's bar code on the identification band, if required.	
——	——	——	19. *Based on facility policy, the third check of the label may occur at this point. If so, recheck the labels with the eMAR/MAR before administering the medications to the patient.*	
——	——	——	20. Put on clean gloves.	
——	——	——	21. Select an appropriate administration site.	
——	——	——	22. Assist the patient to the appropriate position for the site chosen. Drape, as needed, to expose only the site area being used.	
——	——	——	23. *Identify the appropriate landmarks for the site chosen.*	
——	——	——	24. Cleanse the area around the injection site with an antimicrobial swab. Use a firm, circular motion while moving outward from the injection site. Allow the area to dry.	
——	——	——	25. Remove the needle cap by pulling it straight off. Hold the syringe in your dominant hand between the thumb and forefinger.	

Administering an Intramuscular Injection *(Continued)*

Excellent	Satisfactory	Needs Practice		Comments
___	___	___	26. Displace the skin in a Z-track manner. Pull the skin and underlying tissue down or to one side about 1 in (2.5 cm) with your nondominant hand and hold the skin and tissue in this position. Hand and fingers should remain in the appropriate position for the site chosen to continue accurate identification of landmarks and ensure safe injection technique. Alternatively, if, based on assessment of the particular circumstances for an individual patient, the nurse decides not to use the Z-Track technique, the skin should be stretched flat between two fingers and held taut for needle insertion.	
___	___	___	27. Quickly dart the needle into the tissue so that the needle is perpendicular to the patient's body, with the goal of an angle of 90 degrees.	
___	___	___	28. As soon as the needle is in place, use the thumb and forefinger of your nondominant hand to hold the lower end of the syringe, taking care to maintain the displacement of the skin and tissue. Slide your dominant hand to the end of the plunger. Inject the solution slowly (10 sec/mL of medication).	
___	___	___	29. Once the medication has been instilled, wait 10 seconds before withdrawing the needle.	
___	___	___	30. Withdraw the needle smoothly and steadily at the same angle at which it was inserted, supporting tissue around the injection site with your nondominant hand. ***Remove the hand holding the displaced skin and tissue only after removal of the needle.***	
___	___	___	31. Do not recap the used needle. Engage the safety shield or needle guard, if present.	
___	___	___	32. Apply gentle pressure at the site with a dry gauze. ***Do not massage the site.***	
___	___	___	33. Assist the patient to a position of comfort.	
___	___	___	34. Discard the needle and syringe in the appropriate receptacle.	
___	___	___	35. Remove gloves and additional PPE, if used. Perform hand hygiene.	
___	___	___	36. Document the administration of the medication immediately after administration.	
___	___	___	37. Evaluate the patient's response to the medication within the appropriate time frame. Assess site, if possible, within 2 to 4 hours after administration.	

Skills Checklist to Accompany Fundamentals of Nursing:
The Art and Science of Person-Centered Care, 9th edition

Name _____ Date _____

Unit _____ Position _____

Instructor/Evaluator: _____ Position _____

Excellent	Satisfactory	Needs Practice	SKILL 29-8 **Administering Medications by Intravenous Bolus or Push Through an Intravenous Solution**	Comments
			Goal: The prescribed medication is given safely to the patient via the intravenous route.	
——	——	——	1. Gather equipment. Check medication order against the original order in the medical record, according to facility policy. Clarify any inconsistencies. Check the patient's health record for allergies. Check a drug resource to clarify whether the medication needs to be diluted before administration. Check the administration rate.	
——	——	——	2. Know the actions, special nursing considerations, safe dose ranges, purpose of administration, and adverse effects of the medications to be administered. Consider the appropriateness of the medication for this patient.	
——	——	——	3. Perform hand hygiene.	
——	——	——	4. Move the medication supply system to the outside of the patient's room or prepare for administration at the medication supply system in the medication area. Alternatively, access the medication administration supply system at or inside the patient's room.	
——	——	——	5. Unlock the medication supply system or drawer. Enter pass code and scan employee identification, if required.	
——	——	——	6. *Prepare medication for one patient at a time.*	
——	——	——	7. Read the eMAR/MAR and select the proper medication from the medication supply system or the patient's medication drawer.	
——	——	——	8. Compare the label with the eMAR/MAR. Check expiration dates and perform calculations, if necessary. Scan the bar code on the package, if required.	
——	——	——	9. If necessary, withdraw medication from an ampule or vial.	
——	——	——	10. *Depending on facility policy, the third check of the label may occur at this point. If so, when all medications for one patient have been prepared, recheck the labels with the eMAR/MAR before taking the medications to the patient. However, many facilities require the third check to occur at the bedside, after identifying the patient.*	
——	——	——	11. *Lock the medication supply system before leaving it.*	

SKILL 29-8

Administering Medications by Intravenous Bolus or Push Through an Intravenous Solution *(Continued)*

Excellent	Satisfactory	Needs Practice		Comments
——	——	——	12. Transport medications and equipment to the patient's bedside carefully, and keep the medications in sight at all times.	
——	——	——	13. *Ensure that the patient receives the medications at the correct time.*	
——	——	——	14. Perform hand hygiene and put on PPE, if indicated.	
——	——	——	15. *Identify the patient. Compare the information with the eMAR/MAR. The patient should be identified using at least two of the following methods* (The Joint Commission, 2018):	
——	——	——	a. Check the name on the patient's identification band.	
——	——	——	b. Check the identification number on the patient's identification band.	
——	——	——	c. Check the birth date on the patient's identification band.	
——	——	——	d. Ask the patient to state his or her name and birth date, based on facility policy.	
——	——	——	16. Close the door to the room or pull the bedside curtain.	
——	——	——	17. *Complete necessary assessments before administering medications. Check the patient's allergy bracelet or ask the patient about allergies. Explain the purpose and action of the medication to the patient.*	
——	——	——	18. Scan the patient's bar code on the identification band, if required.	
——	——	——	19. *Based on facility policy, the third check of the label may occur at this point. If so, recheck the label with the eMAR/MAR before administering the medications to the patient.*	
——	——	——	20. Assess IV site for presence of inflammation or infiltration or other signs of complications.	
——	——	——	21. If IV infusion is being administered via an infusion pump, pause the pump.	
——	——	——	22. Put on clean gloves.	
——	——	——	23. Select injection port on the administration set that is closest to the patient. Close the clamp on the administration set immediately above the injection port. Do not disconnect the administration set from the venous access device hub (INS, 2016a).	
——	——	——	24. Remove the passive disinfection cap from the needleless connector or end cap on the infusion set injection port. Alternatively, if a passive disinfection cap is not in place, use an antimicrobial swab to vigorously scrub the needleless connector or end cap on the injection port and allow to dry.	

SKILL 29-8

Administering Medications by Intravenous Bolus or Push Through an Intravenous Solution *(Continued)*

Excellent	Satisfactory	Needs Practice		Comments
——	——	——	25. Uncap saline flush syringe. Insert the saline flush syringe into the needleless connector or end cap on the injection port on the administration tubing.	
——	——	——	26. Pull back on the syringe plunger to aspirate the catheter for positive blood return. If positive, instill the solution over 1 minute or flush the line according to facility policy. Remove syringe.	
——	——	——	27. Use an antimicrobial swab to vigorously scrub the needleless connector or end cap on the injection port and allow to dry.	
——	——	——	28. Uncap the medication syringe. Insert the medication syringe into the needleless connector or end cap on the injection port. Using a watch or clock with a second-hand to time the rate, *inject the medication at the recommended rate.*	
——	——	——	29. While administering the medication, observe the infusion site and assess patient for any adverse reaction. If signs of adverse reaction occur, stop infusion immediately and notify the primary health provider.	
——	——	——	30. Detach the medication syringe. Use a new antimicrobial swab to vigorously scrub the needleless connector or end cap on the injection port, and allow to dry. Uncap the second saline flush syringe. Insert the saline flush syringe into the needleless connector or end cap on injection port. Instill the flush solution at the same rate as the administered medication (INS, 2016a).	
——	——	——	31. Remove the flush syringe. Unclamp the administration set above the injection port.	
——	——	——	32. Using an antimicrobial swab, vigorously scrub the needleless connector or end cap on the extension tubing and allow to dry. Attach a passive disinfection cap to the needleless connector or end cap on the extension tubing or the injection port on the administration set.	
——	——	——	33. Restart the infusion pump and check IV fluid infusion rate.	
——	——	——	34. Discard the syringe in the appropriate receptacle.	
——	——	——	35. Remove gloves and additional PPE, if used. Perform hand hygiene.	
——	——	——	36. Document the administration of the medication immediately after administration.	
——	——	——	37. Evaluate the patient's response to the medication within the appropriate time frame.	

Skills Checklist to Accompany Fundamentals of Nursing:
The Art and Science of Person-Centered Care, 9th edition

Name _____ Date _____

Unit _____ Position _____

Instructor/Evaluator: _____ Position _____

SKILL 29-9

Administering a Piggyback Intermittent Intravenous Infusion of Medication

Goal: The medication is delivered safely to the patient via the intravenous route using sterile technique.

Excellent	Satisfactory	Needs Practice		Comments
___	___	___	1. Gather equipment. Check each medication order against the original order in the health record, according to facility policy. Clarify any inconsistencies. Check the patient's health record for allergies.	
___	___	___	2. Know the actions, special nursing considerations, safe dose ranges, purpose of administration, and adverse effects of the medications to be administered. Consider the appropriateness of the medication for this patient. *Assess the compatibility of the ordered medication, diluent, and the infusing IV fluid.*	
___	___	___	3. Perform hand hygiene.	
___	___	___	4. Move the medication supply system to the outside of the patient's room or prepare for administration at the medication supply system in the medication area. Alternatively, access the medication administration supply system at or inside the patient's room.	
___	___	___	5. Unlock the medication supply system or drawer. Enter pass code and scan employee identification, if required.	
___	___	___	6. *Prepare medications for one patient at a time.*	
___	___	___	7. Read the eMAR/MAR and select the proper medication from the medication supply system or the patient's medication drawer.	
___	___	___	8. Compare the label with the eMAR/MAR. Check expiration dates. Confirm the prescribed or appropriate infusion rate. Calculate the drip rate if using a gravity system. Scan the bar code on the package, if required.	
___	___	___	9. *Depending on facility policy, the third check of the label may occur at this point. If so, when all medications for one patient have been prepared, recheck the labels with the eMAR/MAR before taking the medications to the patient. However, many facilities require the third check to occur at the bedside, after identifying the patient.*	
___	___	___	10. *Lock the medication supply system before leaving it.*	
___	___	___	11. Transport medications to the patient's bedside carefully, and keep the medications in sight at all times.	

SKILL 29-9

Administering a Piggyback Intermittent Intravenous Infusion of Medication *(Continued)*

Excellent	Satisfactory	Needs Practice		Comments
——	——	——	12. *Ensure that the patient receives the medications at the correct time.*	
——	——	——	13. Perform hand hygiene and put on PPE, if indicated.	
——	——	——	14. *Identify the patient. Compare the information with the eMAR/MAR. The patient should be identified using at least two of the following methods* (The Joint Commission, 2018):	
——	——	——	a. Check the name on the patient's identification band.	
——	——	——	b. Check the identification number on the patient's identification band.	
——	——	——	c. Check the birth date on the patient's identification band.	
——	——	——	d. Ask the patient to state his or her name and birth date, based on facility policy.	
——	——	——	15. Close the door to the room or pull the bedside curtain.	
——	——	——	16. *Complete necessary assessments before administering medications. Check the patient's allergy bracelet or ask the patient about allergies. Explain the purpose and action of the medication to the patient.*	
——	——	——	17. Scan the patient's bar code on the identification band, if required.	
——	——	——	18. *Based on facility policy, the third check of the label may occur at this point. If so, recheck the labels with the eMAR/MAR before administering the medications to the patient.*	
——	——	——	19. Assess the IV site for the presence of complications.	
——	——	——	20. Close the clamp on the short secondary infusion tubing. Using aseptic technique, remove the cap on the tubing spike and the cap on the port of the medication container, taking care to avoid contaminating either end.	
——	——	——	21. Attach infusion tubing to the medication container by inserting the tubing spike into the port with a firm push and twisting motion, taking care to avoid contaminating either end.	
——	——	——	22. Hang piggyback container on IV pole, positioning it higher than primary IV according to manufacturer's recommendations. If necessary for the particular infusion pump in use, use the metal or plastic hook to lower primary IV fluid container. If using gravity infusion, primary IV fluid container must be lowered.	
——	——	——	23. Place label on administration tubing with the current date.	

SKILL 29-9

Administering a Piggyback Intermittent Intravenous Infusion of Medication *(Continued)*

Excellent	Satisfactory	Needs Practice		Comments
——	——	——	24. Squeeze drip chamber on administration tubing and release. Fill chamber to the line or about half full. Open clamp on administration tubing and prime tubing. Close clamp. Place needleless connector on the end of the tubing, using sterile technique, if required.	
——	——	——	25. Remove the passive disinfection cap from the needleless connector or end cap on the infusion set injection port. Alternatively, if a passive disinfection cap is not in place, use an antimicrobial swab to vigorously scrub the access port or stopcock on the administration set above where the tubing enters the infusion pump or above the roller clamp on the primary IV infusion tubing (gravity infusion).	
——	——	——	26. Connect piggyback setup to the access port or stopcock. If using, turn the stopcock to the open position.	
——	——	——	27. Open clamp on the secondary infusion tubing. Set rate for secondary infusion on infusion pump and begin infusion. If using gravity infusion, use the roller clamp on the primary infusion tubing to regulate the flow at the prescribed delivery rate. Monitor medication infusion at periodic intervals.	
——	——	——	28. Clamp tubing on piggyback set when solution is infused. Follow facility policy regarding disposal of equipment.	
——	——	——	29. Raise primary IV fluid container to original height. *Check primary infusion rate on infusion pump. If using gravity infusion, readjust flow rate of primary IV.*	
——	——	——	30. Remove PPE, if used. Perform hand hygiene.	
——	——	——	31. Document the administration of the medication immediately after administration. Document the volume of fluid administered on the intake and output record, if necessary.	
——	——	——	32. Evaluate the patient's response to the medication within an appropriate time frame. Monitor IV site at periodic intervals.	

Skills Checklist to Accompany Fundamentals of Nursing:
The Art and Science of Person-Centered Care, 9th edition

Name _____ Date _____

Unit _____ Position _____

Instructor/Evaluator: _____ Position _____

Excellent	Satisfactory	Needs Practice	SKILL 29-10 **Administering Medications by Intravenous Bolus or Push Through a Medication or Drug-Infusion Lock** **Goal:** The prescribed medication is given safely to the patient via the intravenous route.	Comments
___	___	___	1. Gather equipment. Check the medication order against the original order in the health record, according to facility policy. Clarify any inconsistencies. Check the patient's health record for allergies. Check a drug resource to clarify whether medication needs to be diluted before bolus administration. Verify the recommended administration rate.	
___	___	___	2. Know the actions, special nursing considerations, safe dose ranges, purpose of administration, and adverse effects of the medications to be administered. Consider the appropriateness of the medication for this patient.	
___	___	___	3. Perform hand hygiene.	
___	___	___	4. Move the medication supply system to the outside of the patient's room or prepare for administration at the medication supply system in the medication area. Alternatively, access the medication administration supply system at or inside the patient's room.	
___	___	___	5. Unlock the medication supply system or drawer. Enter pass code and scan employee identification, if required.	
___	___	___	6. *Prepare medication for one patient at a time.*	
___	___	___	7. Read the eMAR/MAR and select the proper medication from medication supply system or the patient's medication drawer.	
___	___	___	8. Compare the label with the eMAR/MAR. Check expiration dates and perform calculations, if necessary. Scan the bar code on the package, if required.	
___	___	___	9. If necessary, withdraw medication from an ampule or vial.	
___	___	___	10. *Depending on facility policy, the third check of the label may occur at this point. If so, when all medications for one patient have been prepared, recheck the labels with the eMAR/MAR before taking the medications to the patient. However, many facilities require the third check to occur at the bedside, after identifying the patient.*	

SKILL 29-10

Administering Medications by Intravenous Bolus or Push Through a Medication or Drug-Infusion Lock *(Continued)*

Excellent	Satisfactory	Needs Practice		Comments

___ ___ ___	11. *Lock the medication supply system before leaving it.*	
___ ___ ___	12. Transport medications and equipment to the patient's bedside carefully, and keep the medications in sight at all times.	
___ ___ ___	13. *Ensure that the patient receives the medications at the correct time.*	
___ ___ ___	14. Perform hand hygiene and put on PPE, if indicated.	
___ ___ ___	15. *Identify the patient. Compare the information with the eMAR/MAR. The patient should be identified using at least two of the following methods* (The Joint Commission, 2018):	
___ ___ ___	a. Check the name on the patient's identification band.	
___ ___ ___	b. Check the identification number on the patient's identification band.	
___ ___ ___	c. Check the birth date on the patient's identification band.	
___ ___ ___	d. Ask the patient to state his or her name and birth date, based on facility policy.	
___ ___ ___	16. Close the door to the room or pull the bedside curtain.	
___ ___ ___	17. *Complete necessary assessments before administering medications. Check the patient's allergy bracelet or ask the patient about allergies. Explain the purpose and action of the medication to the patient.*	
___ ___ ___	18. Scan the patient's bar code on the identification band, if required.	
___ ___ ___	19. *Based on facility policy, the third check of the label may occur at this point. If so, recheck the labels with the eMAR/MAR before administering the medications to the patient.*	
___ ___ ___	20. Assess IV site for presence of inflammation or infiltration.	
___ ___ ___	21. Put on clean gloves.	
___ ___ ___	22. Remove the passive disinfection cap from the needleless connector or access port of the medication lock. Alternatively, if a passive disinfection cap is not in place, use an antimicrobial swab to vigorously scrub the needleless connector or access port of the medication lock and allow to dry.	
___ ___ ___	23. Uncap saline flush syringe. Stabilize the port with your nondominant hand and insert the saline flush syringe into the needleless connector or end cap on the access port of the medication lock.	

Excellent	Satisfactory	Needs Practice	SKILL 29-10 **Administering Medications by Intravenous Bolus or Push Through a Medication or Drug-Infusion Lock** *(Continued)*	
				Comments
——	——	——	24. Release the clamp on the extension tubing of the medication lock. Pull back on the syringe plunger to aspirate the catheter for positive blood return. If positive, instill the solution over 1 minute or flush the line according to facility policy. Observe the insertion site while inserting the saline. Remove syringe.	
——	——	——	25. Use an antimicrobial swab to vigorously scrub the needleless connector or end cap on the access port of the medication lock and allow to dry.	
——	——	——	26. Uncap the medication syringe. Insert the medication syringe into the needleless connector or end cap on the access port of the medication lock. Using a watch or clock with a second-hand to time the rate, *inject the medication at the recommended rate. Do not force the injection if resistance is felt.*	
——	——	——	27. While administering the medication, observe the infusion site and assess patient for any adverse reaction. If signs of adverse reaction occur, stop infusion immediately and notify the primary health provider.	
——	——	——	28. Remove the medication syringe from the access port. Use a new antimicrobial swab to vigorously scrub the needleless connector or end cap on the access port and allow to dry. Stabilize the port with your nondominant hand. Uncap the second saline flush syringe. Insert the saline flush syringe into the needleless connector or end cap on the access port. Instill the flush solution at the same rate as the administered medication (INS, 2016a).	
——	——	——	29. If the medication lock is capped with positive pressure valve/device, remove syringe, and then clamp the extension tubing. Alternatively, to gain positive pressure if positive pressure valve/device is not present, clamp the extension tubing as you are still flushing the last of the saline into the medication lock. Remove syringe.	
——	——	——	30. Using an antimicrobial swab, vigorously scrub the needleless connector or end cap on the access port of the medication lock and allow to dry. Attach a passive disinfection cap to the needleless connector or end cap on the access port of the medication lock.	
——	——	——	31. Discard the syringe in the appropriate receptacle.	

SKILL 29-10

Administering Medications by Intravenous Bolus or Push Through a Medication or Drug-Infusion Lock *(Continued)*

Excellent	Satisfactory	Needs Practice		Comments
——	——	——	32. Remove gloves and additional PPE, if used. Perform hand hygiene.	
——	——	——	33. Document the administration of the medication immediately after administration.	
——	——	——	34. Evaluate the patient's response to the medication within an appropriate time frame.	

Skills Checklist to Accompany Fundamentals of Nursing:
The Art and Science of Person-Centered Care, 9th edition

Name _____ Date _____

Unit _____ Position _____

Instructor/Evaluator: _____ Position _____

SKILL 30-1

Providing Preoperative Patient Care

Excellent	Satisfactory	Needs Practice	**Goal:** The patient is prepared physically and psychologically to proceed to surgery.	Comments
___	___	___	1. Check the patient's health record for the type of surgery and review the prescribed orders. Review the nursing database, history, and physical examination. Check that the baseline data are recorded; report those that are abnormal.	
___	___	___	2. *Check that all diagnostic testing has been completed and results are available; identify and report abnormal results.* Gather the necessary supplies.	
___	___	___	3. Perform hand hygiene and put on PPE, if indicated.	
___	___	___	4. Identify the patient.	
___	___	___	5. Close the curtains around the bed and close the door to the room, if possible. Explain what you are going to do and why you are going to do it to the patient and significant other. Place necessary supplies on the bedside stand, overbed table, or other surface within easy reach.	
___	___	___	6. Explore the psychological needs of the patient and family related to the surgery.	
___	___	___	a. Establish a therapeutic relationship, encouraging the patient to verbalize concerns or fears.	
___	___	___	b. Use active listening skills, answering questions and clarifying any misinformation.	
___	___	___	c. Use touch, as appropriate, to convey genuine empathy.	
___	___	___	d. Offer to contact spiritual counselor (e.g., priest, minister, rabbi) to meet spiritual needs.	
___	___	___	7. *Identify learning needs of patient and family.* Ensure that the informed consent of the patient for the surgery has been signed, timed, dated, and witnessed. Inquire if the patient has any questions regarding the surgical procedure. Check the patient's record to determine if an advance directive has been completed. If an advance directive has not been completed, discuss with the patient the possibility of completing it, as appropriate. If patient has had surgery before, ask about this experience.	
___	___	___	8. Teach deep-breathing exercises.	

Providing Preoperative Patient Care *(Continued)*

Excellent	Satisfactory	Needs Practice		Comments
——	——	——	9. Teach coughing and splinting.	
——	——	——	10. Teach use of incentive spirometer, as prescribed or indicated.	
——	——	——	11. Teach leg exercises, as appropriate.	
——	——	——	12. Teach about early ambulation, as appropriate.	
——	——	——	13. Assist the patient in putting on graduated compression stockings. Demonstrate how the pneumatic compression device operates.	
——	——	——	14. Teach about turning in the bed.	
——	——	——	a. Instruct the patient to use a pillow or bath blanket to splint where the incision will be. Ask the patient to raise his or her left knee and reach across to grasp the right side rail of the bed). If the patient is turning to the left side, he or she will bend the right knee and grasp the left side rail.	
——	——	——	b. When turning the patient onto the right side, ask the patient to push with bent left leg and pull on the right side rail. Explain to the patient that you will place a pillow behind his/her back to provide support, and that the call bell will be placed within easy reach.	
——	——	——	c. Explain to the patient that position change is recommended every 2 hours.	
——	——	——	15. Provide individualized, developmentally appropriate teaching about pain management options, plans and goals.	
——	——	——	a. Discuss past experiences with pain and interventions that the patient has used to reduce pain.	
——	——	——	b. Discuss the availability of analgesic medication postoperatively.	
——	——	——	c. Discuss the use of PCA, as appropriate.	
——	——	——	d. Explore the use of other alternative and nonpharmacologic methods to reduce pain, such as position change, massage, relaxation/diversion, guided imagery, and meditation.	
——	——	——	16. Review equipment that may be used after surgery.	
——	——	——	a. Show the patient various equipment, such as IV infusion devices, electronic blood pressure cuff, tubes, urinary catheters, and surgical drains.	
——	——	——	17. Provide skin preparation.	
——	——	——	a. *Ask the patient to bathe or shower with the antibacterial soap or solution. Remind the patient to clean the surgical site.*	

SKILL 30-1

Providing Preoperative Patient Care *(Continued)*

Excellent	Satisfactory	Needs Practice		Comments

			18. Provide teaching about and follow dietary/fluid restrictions. *Explain to the patient that both food and fluid will be restricted before surgery to ensure that the stomach contains a minimal amount of gastric secretions. This restriction is important to reduce the risk of aspiration. Emphasize to the patient the importance of avoiding food and fluids during the prescribed time period, because failure to adhere may necessitate cancellation of the surgery.*	
			19. Provide intestinal preparation, as appropriate. In certain situations, such as surgery of the lower gastrointestinal tract, the bowel will need to be prepared by administering enemas or laxatives.	
			a. As needed, explain the purpose of enemas or laxatives before surgery. If the patient will be administered an enema, clarify the steps as needed.	
			20. *Check administration of regularly scheduled medications.* Review with the patient routine medications, over-the-counter medications, and herbal supplements that are taken regularly. Check the medical orders and review with the patient which medications he or she will be permitted to take the day of surgery.	
			21. Provide information to the patient and family regarding timing of surgical events and potential sensations that may be experienced. Explain to patients and their families how long the surgery and postanesthesia care will last, as well as what will be done before, during, and after surgery (e.g., procedures, medications, equipment). Explain to patients that they may not drive themselves home or take public transportation alone if they have had any anesthesia or sedation.	
			22. Remove PPE, if used. Perform hand hygiene.	

Skills Checklist to Accompany Fundamentals of Nursing:
The Art and Science of Person-Centered Care, 9th edition

Name _____ Date _____

Unit _____ Position _____

Instructor/Evaluator: _____ Position _____

SKILL 30-2

Providing Postoperative Care

Goal: The patient recovers from the surgery with postoperative risks minimized by frequent assessments.

Excellent	Satisfactory	Needs Practice		Comments
			Immediate Care	
___	___	___	1. When patient returns from the PACU, participate in hand-off report from the PACU nurse and review the OR and PACU data. Gather the necessary supplies.	
___	___	___	2. Perform hand hygiene and put on PPE, if indicated.	
___	___	___	3. Identify the patient.	
___	___	___	4. Close the curtains around the bed and close the door to the room, if possible. Explain what you are going to do and why you are going to do it to the patient or significant other. Place necessary supplies on the bedside stand, overbed table, or other surface within easy reach.	
___	___	___	5. *Place patient in safe position (semi- or high Fowler's or side-lying). Note level of consciousness.*	
___	___	___	6. *Obtain vital signs. Monitor and record vital signs frequently.* Assessment order may vary, but usual frequency includes taking vital signs every 15 minutes the first hour, every 30 minutes the next 2 hours, every hour for 4 hours, and finally every 4 hours.	
___	___	___	7. Assess the patient's respiratory status. Measure the patient's oxygen saturation level. If oxygen is ordered, ensure accurate delivery device and flow rate.	
___	___	___	8. Assess the patient's cardiovascular status.	
___	___	___	9. Assess the patient's neurovascular status, based on the type of surgery performed.	
___	___	___	10. Provide for warmth, using heated or extra blankets, or forced-air warming device as necessary. Assess skin color and condition.	
___	___	___	11. Put on gloves. Assess the surgical site. Check dressings for color, odor, presence of drains, and amount of drainage. Mark the drainage on the dressing by circling the amount, and include the time. Assess dependent areas, such as turning the patient to assess visually under the patient, for bleeding from the surgical site.	

Providing Postoperative Care *(Continued)*

Excellent	Satisfactory	Needs Practice		Comments

Comments

12. Verify that all tubes and drains are patent and the equipment is working; note the amount of drainage in collection device. If an indwelling urinary catheter is in place, note urinary output.

13. Verify and maintain IV infusion at prescribed rate.

14. Assess for pain. Check health record to verify if analgesic medication was administered in the PACU. Administer analgesics as indicated, prescribed/ordered and appropriate. If the patient has been instructed in the use of PCA for pain management, review its use. Institute nonpharmacologic pain management interventions as appropriate and indicated.

15. Assess for nausea and vomiting. Administer antiemetic medication as indicated, prescribed/ordered, and appropriate.

16. Provide for a safe environment. Keep bed in low position with side rails up, based on facility policy. Have call bell within patient's reach.

17. Remove PPE, if used. Perform hand hygiene.

Ongoing Care

18. Promote optimal respiratory function.
    a. Assess respiratory rate, depth, quality, color, and capillary refill. Ask if the patient is experiencing any difficulty breathing.
    b. Assist with coughing and deep-breathing exercises.
    c. Assist with incentive spirometry, as indicated/ordered.
    d. Assist with early ambulation.
    e. Provide frequent position changes.
    f. Administer oxygen, as ordered.
    g. Monitor pulse oximetry.

19. Promote optimal cardiovascular function:
    a. Assess apical rate, rhythm, and quality and compare with peripheral pulses, color, and blood pressure. Ask if the patient has any chest pains or shortness of breath.
    b. Provide frequent position changes.
    c. Assist with early ambulation.
    d. Apply graduated compression stockings or pneumatic compression devices, if ordered and not in place. If in place, assess for integrity.
    e. Provide leg and range-of-motion exercises if not contraindicated.

Providing Postoperative Care *(Continued)*

Excellent	Satisfactory	Needs Practice		Comments

20. Promote optimal neurologic function:

    a. Assess level of consciousness, movement, and sensation.

    b. Determine the level of orientation to person, place, and time.

    c. Test motor ability by asking the patient to move each extremity.

    d. Evaluate sensation by asking the patient if he or she can feel your touch on an extremity.

21. Promote optimal renal and urinary function and fluid and electrolyte status. Assess intake and output, evaluate for urinary retention and monitor serum electrolyte levels.

    a. Promote voiding by offering bedpan/bedside commode, or assistance to bathroom at regular intervals, noting the frequency, amount, and if any burning or urgency symptoms.

    b. Monitor urinary catheter drainage if present.

    c. Measure intake and output.

22. Promote optimal gastrointestinal function and meet nutritional needs:

    a. Assess abdomen for distention and firmness. Ask if patient feels nauseated, any vomiting, and if passing flatus.

    b. Auscultate for bowel sounds.

    c. Assist with diet progression; encourage fluid intake; monitor intake.

    d. Medicate for nausea and vomiting, as ordered.

23. Promote optimal wound healing.

    a. Assess condition of wound for presence of drains and any drainage.

    b. Use surgical asepsis for dressing changes and drain care.

    c. Inspect all skin surfaces for beginning signs of pressure injury and use pressure-relieving supports to minimize potential skin breakdown.

24. Promote optimal comfort and relief from pain.

    a. Assess for pain (location and intensity using pain scale).

    b. Provide for rest and comfort; provide extra blankets, as needed, for warmth.

    c. Administer analgesics, as needed, and/or initiate non-pharmacologic methods, as appropriate.

Providing Postoperative Care *(Continued)*

Excellent	Satisfactory	Needs Practice		Comments
⎯	⎯	⎯	25. Promote optimal meeting of psychosocial needs:	
⎯	⎯	⎯	a. Provide emotional support to patient and family, as needed.	
⎯	⎯	⎯	b. Explain procedures and offer explanations regarding postoperative recovery, as needed, to both patient and family members.	

Skills Checklist to Accompany Fundamentals of Nursing:
The Art and Science of Person-Centered Care, 9th edition

Name _____ Date _____

Unit _____ Position _____

Instructor/Evaluator: _____ Position _____

Excellent	Satisfactory	Needs Practice	SKILL 31-1 **Providing a Bed Bath**	
			Goal: The patient vocalizes feeling clean and fresh.	**Comments**
——	——	——	1. Review the patient's health record for any limitations in physical activity.	
——	——	——	2. Perform hand hygiene and put on gloves and/or other PPE, if indicated.	
——	——	——	3. Identify the patient. Discuss the procedure with the patient and assess the patient's ability to assist in the bathing process, as well as personal hygiene preferences.	
——	——	——	4. Assemble equipment on the overbed table or other surface within reach.	
——	——	——	5. Close the curtains around the bed and close the door to the room, if possible. Adjust the room temperature, if necessary.	
——	——	——	6. Adjust the bed to a comfortable working height; usually elbow height of the caregiver (VHACEOSH, 2016).	
——	——	——	7. Remove sequential compression devices and antiembolism stockings from lower extremities according to facility protocol.	
——	——	——	8. Put on gloves. Offer the patient a bedpan or urinal.	
——	——	——	9. Remove gloves and perform hand hygiene.	
——	——	——	10. Put on a clean pair of gloves. Lower the side rail nearest to you and assist the patient to the side of bed where you will work. Have the patient lie on his or her back.	
——	——	——	11. Loosen top covers and remove all except the top sheet. Place a bath blanket over the patient and then remove the top sheet while the patient holds the bath blanket in place. If linen is to be reused, fold it over a chair. Place soiled linen in laundry bag. Take care to prevent linen from coming in contact with your clothing.	
——	——	——	12. Remove the patient's gown or clothing and keep the bath blanket in place. If the patient has an IV line and is not wearing a gown with snap sleeves, remove gown from other arm first. Lower the IV container and pass the gown over the tubing and the container. *Rehang the container and check the drip rate.*	

SKILL 31-1
Providing a Bed Bath *(Continued)*

Excellent	Satisfactory	Needs Practice		Comments
——	——	——	13. *Raise side rails.* Fill basin with a sufficient amount of comfortably warm water (100°F to less than 120° to 125°F). Add the skin cleanser, if appropriate, according to manufacturer's directions. Change, as necessary, throughout the bath. Lower side rail nearest to you when you return to the bedside to begin the bath.	
——	——	——	14. Put on gloves, if indicated. Lay a towel across the patient's chest and on top of bath blanket.	
——	——	——	15. With no cleanser on the washcloth, wipe one eye from the inner part of the eye, near the nose, to the outer part. Rinse or turn the cloth before washing the other eye.	
——	——	——	16. Bathe patient's face, neck, and ears. Apply appropriate emollient.	
——	——	——	17. Expose patient's far arm and place towel lengthwise under it. Using firm strokes, wash hand, arm, and axilla, lifting the arm as necessary to access axillary region. Rinse, if necessary, and dry. Apply appropriate emollient. Cover the area with the bath blanket.	
——	——	——	18. Repeat Action 17 for the arm nearest you. Another option might be to bathe one side of the patient first and then move to the other side of the bed to complete the bath.	
——	——	——	19. Spread a towel across patient's chest. Lower bath blanket to patient's umbilical area. Wash, rinse, if necessary, and dry chest. Keep chest covered with towel between the wash and rinse. Pay special attention to the folds of skin under the breasts. Apply appropriate emollient.	
——	——	——	20. Lower bath blanket to the perineal area. Place a towel over patient's chest.	
——	——	——	21. Wash, rinse, if necessary, and dry abdomen. Carefully inspect and clean umbilical area and any abdominal folds or creases. Apply appropriate emollient.	
——	——	——	22. Return bath blanket to original position and expose far leg. Place towel under far leg. Using firm strokes, wash, rinse, if necessary, and dry leg from ankle to knee and knee to groin. Apply appropriate emollient.	
——	——	——	23. Wash, rinse if necessary, and dry the foot. Pay particular attention to the areas between toes. Apply appropriate emollient.	
——	——	——	24. Repeat Actions 22 and 23 for the other leg and foot.	
——	——	——	25. Make sure patient is covered with bath blanket. Change water and washcloth at this point or earlier, if necessary.	

Excellent	Satisfactory	Needs Practice		SKILL 31-1 **Providing a Bed Bath** *(Continued)*	
					Comments
——	——	——	26.	Assist patient to a prone or side-lying position. Put on gloves, if not applied earlier. Position bath blanket and towel to expose only the back and buttocks.	
——	——	——	27.	Wash, rinse, if necessary, and dry back and buttocks area. *Pay particular attention to cleansing between gluteal folds, and observe for any redness or skin breakdown in the sacral area.*	
——	——	——	28.	If not contraindicated, give patient a backrub. Alternatively, back massage may be given after perineal care. Apply appropriate emollient and/or skin barrier product.	
——	——	——	29.	Raise the side rail. Refill basin with clean water. Discard washcloth and towel. Remove gloves and put on clean gloves.	
——	——	——	30.	Clean perineal area or set patient up so that he or she can complete perineal self-care. If the patient is unable to do so, lower the side rail and complete perineal care. Follow the guidelines in the Guidelines for Nursing Care 31-1 earlier in the chapter. Apply skin barrier, as indicated. Raise side rail, remove gloves, and perform hand hygiene.	
——	——	——	31.	Help patient put on a clean gown or clothing and assist with the use of other personal toiletries, such as deodorant or cosmetics.	
——	——	——	32.	Protect pillow with towel, and groom patient's hair.	
——	——	——	33.	*When finished, make sure the patient is comfortable, with the side rails up and the bed in the lowest position.*	
——	——	——	34.	Change bed linens. Dispose of soiled linens according to facility policy. Clean bath basin according to facility policy before returning to storage at bedside. Remove gloves and any other PPE, if used. Perform hand hygiene.	

Skills Checklist to Accompany Fundamentals of Nursing:
The Art and Science of Person-Centered Care, 9th edition

Name _____   Date _____

Unit _____   Position _____

Instructor/Evaluator: _____   Position _____

Excellent	Satisfactory	Needs Practice	SKILL 31-2 **Assisting the Patient With Oral Care**	Comments
			Goal: The patient has a clean mouth and clean teeth, exhibits a positive body image, and verbalizes the importance of oral care.	
___	___	___	1. Perform hand hygiene and put on gloves if assisting with oral care, and/or other PPE, if indicated.	
___	___	___	2. Identify the patient. Explain the procedure to the patient.	
___	___	___	3. Assemble equipment on overbed table or other surface within patient's reach.	
___	___	___	4. Close the room door or curtains. Place the bed at an appropriate and comfortable working height; usually elbow height of the caregiver (VHACEOSH, 2016).	
___	___	___	5. Lower side rail and assist the patient to a sitting position, if permitted, or turn the patient onto side. Place towel across the patient's chest.	
___	___	___	6. Encourage the patient to brush own teeth according to the following guidelines. Assist, if necessary.	
___	___	___	a. Moisten toothbrush and apply toothpaste to bristles.	
___	___	___	b. Place brush at a 45-degree angle to gum line and brush from gum line to crown of each tooth. Brush outer and inner surfaces. Brush back and forth across biting surface of each tooth.	
___	___	___	c. Brush tongue gently with toothbrush.	
___	___	___	d. Have patient rinse vigorously with water and spit into emesis basin. Repeat until clear. Suction may be used as an alternative for removal of fluid and secretions from the mouth.	

Excellent	Satisfactory	Needs Practice		Comments
——	——	——	7. Assist patient to floss teeth, if appropriate:	
——	——	——	a. Remove approximately 18 in of dental floss from container or use a plastic floss holder. Wrap most of the floss around one of the middle fingers. Wind the remaining floss around the same finger of the opposite hand, keeping about 1 to 1.5 in of floss taut between the fingers.	
——	——	——	b. Insert floss gently between teeth, moving it back and forth downward to the gums.	
——	——	——	c. Move the floss up and down, first on one side of a tooth and then on the side of the other tooth, until the surfaces are clean. Repeat in the spaces between all teeth and the backside of the last teeth.	
——	——	——	d. Instruct patient to rinse mouth well with water after flossing.	
——	——	——	8. Offer a mouth rinse if patient prefers or if use has been recommended.	
——	——	——	9. Offer lip balm or petroleum jelly.	
——	——	——	10. Remove equipment. Remove gloves and discard. Raise side rail and lower bed. Assist patient to a position of comfort.	
——	——	——	11. Remove any other PPE, if used. Perform hand hygiene.	

Skills Checklist to Accompany Fundamentals of Nursing:
The Art and Science of Person-Centered Care, 9th edition

Name _____   Date _____

Unit _____   Position _____

Instructor/Evaluator: _____   Position _____

SKILL 31-3

Providing Oral Care for the Dependent Patient

Goal: The patient's mouth and teeth are clean; the patient does not experience impaired oral mucous membranes; the patient demonstrates improvement in body image; and the patient verbalizes, if able, an understanding about the importance of oral care.

Excellent	Satisfactory	Needs Practice		Comments
____	____	____	1. Perform hand hygiene and put on PPE, if indicated.	
____	____	____	2. Identify the patient. Explain the procedure to the patient.	
____	____	____	3. Assemble equipment on overbed table or other surface within reach.	
____	____	____	4. Close the room door or curtains. Place the bed at an appropriate and comfortable working height, usually elbow height of the caregiver (VHACEOSH, 2016). Lower one side rail and position the patient on the side, with head tilted forward. Place towel across the patient's chest and emesis basin in position under chin. Depending on equipment in use, connect the suction toothbrush or suction catheter to suction tubing and turn on suction. Put on gloves.	
____	____	____	5. Gently open the patient's mouth by applying pressure to the lower jaw at the front of the mouth. Do not use fingers to hold the patient's mouth open. Use another toothbrush or mouth prop to keep the mouth open (Johnson, 2011). Remove dentures, if present.	
____	____	____	6. If using a regular toothbrush and suction catheter, one care giver provides oral cleaning and the other removes secretions with the suction catheter.	
____	____	____	7. Brush the teeth and gums carefully with toothbrush and paste or other oral cleanser. Lightly brush the tongue.	
____	____	____	8. Moisten toothbrush with water to rinse the oral cavity. *Position patient's head to allow for return of water. If using regular toothbrush, use suction catheter to remove the water and cleanser from oral cavity.*	
____	____	____	9. Using the suction swab, apply a therapeutic antiseptic mouth rinse as indicated. Apply oral moisturizer as indicated.	
____	____	____	10. Clean the dentures before replacing.	
____	____	____	11. Apply lubricant to patient's lips.	
____	____	____	12. Remove equipment and return patient to a position of comfort. Remove gloves. Raise side rail and lower bed.	
____	____	____	13. Remove additional PPE, if used. Perform hand hygiene.	

Skills Checklist to Accompany Fundamentals of Nursing:
The Art and Science of Person-Centered Care, 9th edition

Name _____ Date _____

Unit _____ Position _____

Instructor/Evaluator: _____ Position _____

SKILL 31-4

Making an Unoccupied Bed

Excellent	Satisfactory	Needs Practice		Comments
			Goal: The bed linens are changed without injury to the nurse or patient.	
___	___	___	1. Perform hand hygiene. Put on PPE, as indicated.	
___	___	___	2. Explain to the patient what you are going to do and the reason for doing it, if the patient is present in room.	
___	___	___	3. Assemble necessary equipment on the bedside stand, overbed table, or other surface within reach.	
___	___	___	4. Adjust the bed to a comfortable working height, usually elbow height of the caregiver (VHACEOSH, 2016). Drop the side rails.	
___	___	___	5. Disconnect call bell or any tubes from bed linens.	
___	___	___	6. Put on gloves. Loosen all linen as you move around the bed, from the head of the bed on the far side to the head of the bed on the near side.	
___	___	___	7. Fold reusable linens, such as sheets, blankets, or spread, in place on the bed in fourths and hang them over a clean chair.	
___	___	___	8. Snugly roll all the soiled linen inside the bottom sheet. Hold linen away from your body and place directly into the laundry hamper. *Do not place on floor or furniture. Do not hold soiled linens against your clothing.*	
___	___	___	9. If possible, shift mattress up to head of bed. If mattress is soiled, clean and dry according to facility policy before applying new sheets.	
___	___	___	10. Remove your gloves, unless indicated for transmission-based precautions. Place the bottom sheet on the mattress and secure the bottom sheet over the corners at the head and foot of the mattress.	
___	___	___	11. Push the sheet open to the center of the mattress, pulling the sheet taut from the secured corners.	

SKILL 31-4

Making an Unoccupied Bed *(Continued)*

Excellent	Satisfactory	Needs Practice		Comments

___	___	___	12. If using, place the drawsheet with its centerfold in the center of the bed and positioned so it will be located under the patient's midsection. Open the drawsheet and fan-fold to the center of the mattress. If a protective pad is used, place it over the drawsheet in the proper area and open to the centerfold. Not all facilities use drawsheets routinely. The nurse may decide to use one. In some institutions, the protective pad doubles as a drawsheet. Tuck the drawsheet securely under the mattress.	
___	___	___	13. Move to the other side of the bed to secure bottom linens. Pull the bottom sheet tightly and secure over the corners at the head and foot of the mattress. Pull the drawsheet tightly and tuck it securely under the mattress.	
___	___	___	14. Place the top sheet on the bed with its centerfold in the center of the bed and with the hem even with the head of the mattress. Unfold the top sheet. Follow same procedure with top blanket or spread, placing the upper edge about 6 in below the top of the sheet.	
___	___	___	15. Tuck the top sheet and blanket under the foot of the bed on the near side. Miter the corners.	
___	___	___	16. Fold the upper 6 in of the top sheet down over the spread and make a cuff.	
___	___	___	17. Move to the other side of the bed and follow the same procedure for securing top sheets under the foot of the bed and making a cuff.	
___	___	___	18. Place the pillows on the bed. Open each pillowcase in the same manner as you opened other linens. Gather the pillowcase over one hand toward the closed end. Grasp the pillow with the hand inside the pillowcase. Keep a firm hold on the top of the pillow and pull the cover onto the pillow. Place the pillow at the head of the bed.	
___	___	___	19. Fan-fold or pie-fold the top linens.	
___	___	___	20. Secure the signal device on the bed, according to facility policy.	
___	___	___	21. Raise the side rail and lower the bed.	
___	___	___	22. Dispose of soiled linen according to facility policy.	
___	___	___	23. Remove any other PPE, if used. Perform hand hygiene.	

Skills Checklist to Accompany Fundamentals of Nursing:
The Art and Science of Person-Centered Care, 9th edition

Name _____ Date _____

Unit _____ Position _____

Instructor/Evaluator: _____ Position _____

Excellent	Satisfactory	Needs Practice		Comments
			SKILL 31-5 **Making an Occupied Bed** **Goal:** The bed linens are applied without injury to the patient or nurse.	
——	——	——	1. Check health care record for limitations on patient's physical activity.	
——	——	——	2. Perform hand hygiene. Put on PPE, as indicated.	
——	——	——	3. Identify the patient. Explain what you are going to do.	
——	——	——	4. Assemble equipment on overbed table or other surface within reach.	
——	——	——	5. Close the curtains around the bed and close the door to the room, if possible.	
——	——	——	6. Adjust the bed to a comfortable working height, usually elbow height of the caregiver (VHACEOSH, 2016).	
——	——	——	7. Lower side rail nearest you, leaving the opposite side rail up. Place bed in flat position unless contraindicated.	
——	——	——	8. Put on gloves. Check bed linens for patient's personal items. *Disconnect the call bell or any tubes/drains from bed linens.*	
——	——	——	9. Place a bath blanket over the patient. Have the patient hold on to bath blanket while you reach under it and remove top linens. Leave top sheet in place if a bath blanket is not used. Fold linen that is to be reused over the back of a chair. Discard soiled linen in laundry bag or hamper. *Do not place on floor or furniture. Do not hold soiled linens against your clothing.*	
——	——	——	10. If possible, and another person is available to assist, grasp mattress securely and shift it up to head of bed.	
——	——	——	11. Assist patient to turn toward opposite side of the bed, and reposition pillow under patient's head.	
——	——	——	12. Loosen all bottom linens from head, foot, and side of bed.	
——	——	——	13. Fan-fold or roll soiled linens as close to the patient as possible.	
——	——	——	14. Use clean linen and make the near side of the bed. Place the bottom sheet in the center of the bed. Open the sheet and pull the bottom sheet over the corners at the head and foot of the mattress. Push the sheet toward the center of the bed, pulling it taut and positioning it under the old linens.	

SKILL 31-5

Making an Occupied Bed *(Continued)*

Excellent	Satisfactory	Needs Practice		Comments

15. If using, place the drawsheet with its centerfold in the center of the bed and positioned so it will be located under the patient's midsection. Open the drawsheet and fan-fold it to the center of the mattress. Tuck the drawsheet securely under the mattress. If a protective pad is used, place it over the drawsheet in the proper area and open to the centerfold. Not all facilities use drawsheets routinely. The nurse may decide to use one.

16. Raise side rail. Assist patient to roll over the folded linen in the middle of the bed toward you. Reposition pillow and bath blanket or top sheet. Move to other side of the bed and lower side rail.

17. Loosen and remove all bottom linen. Discard soiled linen in laundry bag or hamper. ***Do not place on floor or furniture. Do not hold soiled linens against your clothing.***

18. Ease clean linen from under the patient. Pull the bottom sheet taut and secure at the corners at the head and foot of the mattress. Pull the drawsheet tight and smooth. Tuck the drawsheet securely under the mattress.

19. Assist patient to turn back to the center of bed. Remove pillow and change pillowcase. Open each pillowcase in the same manner as you opened other linens. Gather the pillowcase over one hand toward the closed end. Grasp the pillow with the hand inside the pillowcase. Keep a firm hold on the top of the pillow and pull the cover onto the pillow. Place the pillow under the patient's head.

20. Apply top linen, sheet, and blanket, if desired, so that it is centered. Fold the top linens over at the patient's shoulders to make a cuff. Have patient hold on to top linen and remove the bath blanket from underneath.

21. Secure top linens under foot of mattress and miter corners. Loosen top linens over patient's feet by grasping them in the area of the feet and pulling gently toward foot of bed.

22. Return patient to a position of comfort. Remove your gloves. Raise side rail and lower bed. Reattach call bell.

23. Dispose of soiled linens according to facility policy.

24. Remove any other PPE, if used. Perform hand hygiene.

Skills Checklist to Accompany Fundamentals of Nursing:
The Art and Science of Person-Centered Care, 9th edition

Name _____ Date _____

Unit _____ Position _____

Instructor/Evaluator: _____ Position _____

SKILL 32-1
Preventing Pressure Injury

Excellent	Satisfactory	Needs Practice	**Goal:** The patient does not develop a pressure injury.	Comments
____	____	____	1. Perform hand hygiene and put on PPE, if indicated.	
____	____	____	2. Identify the patient.	
____	____	____	3. Discuss pressure injury prevention with the patient and/or patient caregivers. Explain what pressure injury is, the causes of pressure injuries, and the importance of a pressure injury prevention plan (WOCN, 2016).	
____	____	____	4. Assess the patient's skin at least daily, paying special attention to the skin over bony prominences and the skin in contact with medical devices (Doughty & McNichol, 2016; NPUAP, EPUAT, PPPIA, 2014a).	
____	____	____	5. Assess the patient's risk for pressure injury upon entry to a health care setting and on a regularly scheduled basis or when there is a significant change in the patient's condition, incorporating appropriate assessment tools and scales, based on facility policy (WOCN, 2016).	
____	____	____	6. Utilize appropriate support surfaces to redistribute tissue loads, based on facility policy and availability. Appropriate support surfaces may include, but are not limited to, integrated bed systems, specialized and/or low-pressure mattresses and overlays, seating surfaces and cushions, heel elevation devices, and foam positioning wedges.	
____	____	____	Note: Pressure redistribution devices should serve as adjuncts and not replacements for repositioning of patients (WOCN, 2016). ***Do not use foam rings, foam cut-outs, or donut-type devices.*** The Wound, Ostomy and Continence Nurses Society (WOCN, 2016) has developed a content-validated algorithm for support surface selection.	
____	____	____	7. Routinely reposition the patient; at least every 2 hours for bedridden patients and every hour for patients in a chair or wheelchair (Doughty & McNichol, 2016). Consider the pressure redistribution support surface in use as well as the individual patient's status when determining the frequency of repositioning; the use of some types of support surfaces may extend the frequency (Doughty & McNichol; NPUAP, EPUAP, PPPIA, 2014a).	

Excellent	Satisfactory	Needs Practice	

Preventing Pressure Injury *(Continued)*

Comments

——	——	——	Note: Regular repositioning may not be possible due to the patient's medical condition and alternative strategies such as a "high-specification bed" may be required (NPUAP, EPUAP, PPPIA, 2014a; WOCN, 2016.)
——	——	——	8. Use a 30-degree side-lying position (lateral tilt position) when positioning patients at risk for pressure injury in side-lying positions (WOCN, 2016).
——	——	——	9. Encourage and provide early mobilization. Develop a schedule for progressive sitting and ambulation as rapidly as tolerated by the individual patient. Collaborate with the physical and occupational therapists to develop an individualized intervention plan.
——	——	——	10. Maintain the head-of-bed elevation at or below 30 degrees, or at the lowest degree of elevation appropriate for the patient's medical condition.
——	——	——	11. Consider the use of a prophylactic dressing, such as a polyurethane foam dressing, on bony prominences, such as heels and the sacrum. Replace prophylactic dressings that are damaged, displaced, loosened or excessively moist (NPUAP, EPUAP, PPPIA, 2014a).
——	——	——	12. Consider the use of low-friction patient care textiles, such as bed linens and patient gowns, and the use of silk-like fabrics instead of cotton or cotton-blend fabrics.
——	——	——	13. Utilize proper lifting, positioning, and repositioning techniques (safe patient handling and movement techniques); for example, use lift/repositioning sheets and sufficient caregivers when moving a patient. Collaborate with the physical and occupational therapists to develop an individualized intervention plan.
——	——	——	14. Utilize interventions to protect the skin from excessive exposure to moisture from wound exudate, perspiration, mucus, saliva, fistula and stoma effluent, and urinary and fecal incontinence.
——	——	——	15. Provide appropriate interventions to support the patient's nutritional status and ensure adequate intake. Interventions may include strategies to enhance oral intake, nutritional supplements, fortified foods, and/or enteral or parenteral feeding (Baranoski & Ayello, 2016). Collaborate with the registered dietician and dietary staff to develop an individualized nutrition intervention plan (NPUAP, EPUAP, PPPIA, 2014a).

Excellent	Satisfactory	Needs Practice		Comments
——	——	——	16. Implement interventions to prevent pressure injury related to the use of medical devices, based on the individual patient's situation.	
——	——	——	a. Ensure correct for patient size and application of devices in use.	
——	——	——	b. Use cushioning dressings under the device, as appropriate to the individual patient and clinical use (NPUAP, EPUAP, PPPIA, 2014a).	
——	——	——	c. Inspect the skin under the devices and observe for edema under the devices at least twice daily or more often, as indicated.	
——	——	——	d. Remove device as soon as medically feasible. Reposition or rotate any medical device daily when possible.	
——	——	——	e. Keep the skin clean and dry under medical devices.	
——	——	——	17. Provide education to the patient and caregiver(s) about the prevention plan and ways to minimize the risk of pressure injury.	
——	——	——	18. Remove gloves and additional PPE, if used. Perform hand hygiene.	
——	——	——	19. Evaluate the patient's response to interventions. Reassess and alter care plan as indicated by facility policies and procedures, as appropriate.	

Skills Checklist to Accompany Fundamentals of Nursing:
The Art and Science of Person-Centered Care, 9th edition

Name _____ Date _____

Unit _____ Position _____

Instructor/Evaluator: _____ Position _____

Excellent	Satisfactory	Needs Practice	SKILL 32-2 **Cleaning a Wound and Applying a Dressing (General Guidelines)**	Comments
			Goal: The wound is cleaned and a dressing is applied without contaminating the wound area, causing trauma to the wound, or causing the patient to experience pain or discomfort.	
____	____	____	1. Review the patient's health record for prescribed wound care or the nursing care plan related to wound care. Gather necessary supplies.	
____	____	____	2. Perform hand hygiene and put on PPE, if indicated.	
____	____	____	3. Identify the patient.	
____	____	____	4. Assemble equipment on the overbed table or other surface within reach.	
____	____	____	5. Close the curtains around the bed and close the door to the room, if possible. Explain to the patient what you are going to do and why you are going to do it.	
____	____	____	6. Assess the patient for the possible need for nonpharmacologic pain-reducing interventions or analgesic medication before wound care dressing change. Administer appropriate prescribed analgesic. Allow enough time for the analgesic to achieve its effectiveness.	
____	____	____	7. Place a waste receptacle or bag at a convenient location for use during the procedure.	
____	____	____	8. Adjust the bed to a comfortable working height, usually elbow height of the caregiver (VHACEOSH, 2016).	
____	____	____	9. Assist the patient to a comfortable position that provides easy access to the wound area. Use the bath blanket to cover any exposed area other than the wound. Place a waterproof pad under the wound site.	
____	____	____	10. Check the position of drains, tubes, or other adjuncts before removing the dressing. Put on clean, disposable gloves and loosen the tape or adhesive edge on the old dressings by removing in the direction of hair growth and the use of a push–pull method. Push–pull method: lift a corner of the dressing away from the skin, and then gently push the skin away from the dressing/adhesive. Continue moving fingers of the opposite hand to support the skin as the product is removed (McNichol et al., 2013). Carefully lift the adhesive barrier from the surrounding skin to prevent medical adhesive–related skin injury (MARSI). Remove the sides/edges first, then the center. If there is resistance, use an adhesive remover (McNichol et al., 2013).	

Cleaning a Wound and Applying a Dressing
(General Guidelines) *(Continued)*

Excellent	Satisfactory	Needs Practice		Comments

___ ___ ___			11. Carefully remove the soiled dressings. If any part of the dressing sticks to the underlying skin, use small amounts of sterile saline to help loosen and remove it.
___ ___ ___			12. After removing the dressing, note the presence, amount, type, color, and odor of any drainage on the dressings. Place soiled dressings in the appropriate waste receptacle. Remove your gloves and dispose of them in an appropriate waste receptacle.
___ ___ ___			13. Perform hand hygiene.
___ ___ ___			14. Inspect the wound site for size, appearance, and drainage. Assess if any pain is present. Check the status of sutures, adhesive closure strips, staples, and drains or tubes, if present. Note any problems to include in your documentation.
___ ___ ___			15. *Using sterile technique, prepare a sterile work area and open the needed supplies.*
___ ___ ___			16. Open the sterile cleaning solution. Depending on the amount of cleaning needed, the solution might be poured directly over gauze sponges over a container for small cleaning jobs, or into a basin for more complex or larger cleaning.
___ ___ ___			17. Put on sterile gloves. Alternatively, clean gloves (clean technique) may be used when cleaning a chronic wound or pressure injury.
___ ___ ___			18. Clean the wound. *Clean from top to bottom and/or from the center to the outside.* Use new gauze for each wipe, placing the used gauze in the waste receptacle. Alternatively, spray the wound from top to bottom with a commercially prepared wound cleanser; wound irrigation is often used to clean open wounds and may also be used for other types of wounds.
___ ___ ___			19. Once the wound is cleaned, dry the area using a gauze sponge in the same manner.
___ ___ ___			20. If a drain is in use at the wound location, clean around the drain.
___ ___ ___			21. Remove gloves and place in the waste receptacle. Perform hand hygiene.

Cleaning a Wound and Applying a Dressing (General Guidelines) *(Continued)*

Excellent	Satisfactory	Needs Practice		Comments
——	——	——	22. Put on sterile gloves. Alternately, clean gloves (clean technique) may be used when cleaning a chronic wound or pressure injury. Apply a skin protectant or barrier to the healthy skin around the wound where the dressing adhesive or tape will be placed and where wound drainage may come in contact with the skin.	
——	——	——	23. Apply any topical medications, foams, gels, and/or gauze to the wound as prescribed; ensure products stay confined to the wound and do not impact on intact surrounding tissue/skin.	
——	——	——	24. Gently place a layer of dry, sterile dressing or other prescribed cover dressing at the wound center and extend it at least 1 in beyond the wound in all directions. Alternately, follow the manufacturer's directions for application. Forceps may be used to apply the dressing.	
——	——	——	25. As necessary, apply a surgical or abdominal pad (ABD) over the gauze at the site of the outermost layer of the dressing, with the side of the dressing with the blue line facing away from the patient. Alternately, note the side of the dressing that contains the moisture barrier and place away from the patient, based on the dressing material in use.	
——	——	——	Note: May not be necessary or appropriate, based on the cover dressing used in step 22.	
——	——	——	26. Apply tape, Montgomery straps, or roller gauze to secure the dressings. Alternately, many commercial wound products are self-adhesive and do not require additional tape. Remove and discard gloves.	
——	——	——	27. After securing the dressing, label it with date and time. Remove all remaining equipment; place the patient in a comfortable position, with side rails up as indicated and bed in the lowest position.	
——	——	——	28. Remove PPE, if used. Perform hand hygiene.	
——	——	——	29. Check all wound dressings at least every shift. More frequent checks may be needed if the wound is more complex or dressings become saturated quickly.	

Skills Checklist to Accompany Fundamentals of Nursing:
The Art and Science of Person-Centered Care, 9th edition

Name _____ Date _____

Unit _____ Position _____

Instructor/Evaluator: _____ Position _____

SKILL 32-3
Performing Irrigation of a Wound

Goal: The wound is cleaned without contamination or trauma and without causing the patient to experience pain or discomfort.

Columns: Excellent | Satisfactory | Needs Practice | | Comments

1. Review the patient's health record for prescribed wound care or the nursing care plan related to wound care. Gather necessary supplies.

2. Perform hand hygiene and put on PPE, if indicated.

3. Identify the patient.

4. Assemble equipment on the overbed table or other surface within reach.

5. Close the curtains around the bed and close the door to the room if possible. Explain what you are going to do and why you are going to do it to the patient.

6. Assess the patient for possible need for nonpharmacologic pain-reducing interventions or analgesic medication before wound care and/or dressing change. Administer appropriate prescribed analgesic. Allow enough time for the analgesic to achieve its effectiveness before beginning the procedure.

7. Place a waste receptacle or bag at a convenient location for use during the procedure.

8. Adjust the bed to a comfortable working height, usually elbow height of the caregiver (VHACEOSH, 2016).

9. Assist the patient to a comfortable position that provides easy access to the wound area. Position the patient so the irrigation solution will flow from the clean end of the wound toward the dirtier end or top to bottom. Use the bath blanket to cover any exposed area other than the wound. Place a waterproof pad under the wound site.

10. Put on a gown, mask, and eye protection or face shield.

11. Check the position of drains, tubes, or other adjuncts before removing the dressing. Put on clean, disposable gloves and loosen the tape on the old dressings by removing in the direction of hair growth and the use of a push–pull method. Push–pull method: lift a corner of the dressing away from the skin, then gently push the skin away from the dressing/adhesive. Continue moving fingers of the opposite hand to support the skin as the product is

Performing Irrigation of a Wound (Continued)

Excellent	Satisfactory	Needs Practice		Comments
			removed (McNichol et al., 2013). Carefully lift the adhesive barrier from the surrounding skin to prevent medical adhesive–related skin injury (MARSI). Remove the sides/edges first, then the center. If there is resistance, use an adhesive remover (McNichol et al., 2013).	
___	___	___	12. Carefully remove the soiled dressings. If any part of the dressing sticks to the underlying skin, use small amounts of sterile saline to help loosen and remove it.	
___	___	___	13. After removing the dressing, note the presence, amount, type, color, and odor of any drainage on the dressings. Place soiled dressings in the appropriate waste receptacle.	
___	___	___	14. Assess the wound for appearance, stage, presence of eschar, granulation tissue, epithelialization, undermining, tunneling, necrosis, sinus tract, and drainage. Assess the appearance of the surrounding tissue. Measure the wound.	
___	___	___	15. Remove your gloves and put them in the receptacle. Perform hand hygiene.	
___	___	___	16. Set up a sterile field, if indicated, and wound cleaning and irrigation supplies. Pour warmed sterile irrigating solution into the sterile container. Put on the sterile gloves. Alternately, clean gloves (clean technique) may be used when cleaning a chronic wound or pressure injury.	
___	___	___	17. Position the sterile basin below the wound to collect the irrigation fluid.	
___	___	___	18. Fill the irrigation syringe with solution. Alternately, irrigation solution may be packaged in individual, single-use syringe; remove cap on syringe. *Using your nondominant hand,* gently apply pressure to the basin against the skin below the wound to form a seal with the skin.	
___	___	___	19. *Direct a stream of solution into the wound. Keep the tip of the syringe at least 1 in above the upper edge of the wound. Flush all wound areas.*	
___	___	___	20. Watch for the solution to flow smoothly and evenly. When the solution from the wound flows out clear, discontinue irrigation.	
___	___	___	21. Once the wound is cleaned, dry the surrounding skin using a gauze sponge.	
___	___	___	22. If a drain is in use at the wound location, clean around the drain.	

Excellent	Satisfactory	Needs Practice		
			SKILL 32-3	
			Performing Irrigation of a Wound *(Continued)*	
				Comments
——	——	——	23. Remove gloves and place in a waste receptacle. Perform hand hygiene.	
——	——	——	24. Put on sterile gloves. Alternately, clean gloves (clean technique) may be used when cleaning a chronic wound or pressure injury. Apply a skin protectant or barrier to the healthy skin around the wound where the dressing adhesive or tape will be placed and where wound drainage may come in contact with skin.	
——	——	——	25. Apply any topical medications, foams, gels, and/or gauze to the wound as prescribed; ensure products stay confined to the wound and do not impact on intact surrounding tissue/skin.	
——	——	——	26. Gently place a layer of dry, sterile dressing or other prescribed cover dressing at the wound center and extend it at least 1 in beyond the wound in all directions. Alternately, follow the manufacturer's directions for application. Forceps may be used to apply the dressing.	
——	——	——	27. Apply tape, Montgomery straps, or roller gauze to secure the dressings, if needed. Alternately, many commercial wound products are self-adhesive and do not require additional tape. Remove and discard gloves.	
——	——	——	28. After securing the dressing, label it with date and time. Remove all remaining equipment; place the patient in a comfortable position, with side rails up as indicated and bed in the lowest position.	
——	——	——	29. Remove PPE, if used. Perform hand hygiene.	
——	——	——	30. Check all wound dressings at least every shift. More frequent checks may be needed if the wound is more complex or dressings become saturated quickly.	

Skills Checklist to Accompany Fundamentals of Nursing:
The Art and Science of Person-Centered Care, 9th edition

Name _____   Date _____

Unit _____   Position _____

Instructor/Evaluator: _____   Position _____

SKILL 32-4

Caring for a Jackson–Pratt Drain

Goal: The drain is patent and intact.

Excellent	Satisfactory	Needs Practice		Comments
____	____	____	1. Review the patient's health record for prescribed wound care or the nursing care plan related to wound/drain care. Gather necessary supplies.	
____	____	____	2. Perform hand hygiene and put on PPE, if indicated.	
____	____	____	3. Identify the patient.	
____	____	____	4. Assemble equipment on the overbed table or other surface within reach.	
____	____	____	5. Close the curtains around the bed and close the door to the room, if possible. Explain what you are going to do and why you are going to do it to the patient.	
____	____	____	6. Assess the patient for possible need for nonpharmacologic pain-reducing interventions or analgesic medication before wound care dressing change. Administer appropriate prescribed analgesic. Allow enough time for the analgesic to achieve its effectiveness before beginning the procedure.	
____	____	____	7. Place a waste receptacle at a convenient location for use during the procedure.	
____	____	____	8. Adjust the bed to a comfortable working height, usually elbow height of the caregiver (VHACEOSH, 2016).	
____	____	____	9. Assist the patient to a comfortable position that provides easy access to the drain and/or wound area. Use a bath blanket to cover any exposed area other than the drain. Place a waterproof pad under the drain site.	
____	____	____	10. Put on clean gloves; put on mask or face shield, as indicated.	
____	____	____	11. Using sterile technique, open a gauze pad, making a sterile field with the outer wrapper.	
____	____	____	12. Place the graduated collection container under the drain outlet. Without contaminating the outlet valve, pull off the cap. The chamber will expand completely as it draws in air. *Empty the chamber's contents completely into the container. Use the gauze pad to wipe the outlet. Fully compress the chamber with one hand and replace the cap with your other hand.*	

Excellent	Satisfactory	Needs Practice		Comments

—— —— —— 13. Check the patency of the equipment. Bulb should remain compressed. *Check that the tubing is free from twists and kinks.*

—— —— —— 14. Secure the JP drain to the patient's gown below the wound with a safety pin, *making sure that there is no tension on the tubing.*

—— —— —— 15. Carefully measure and record the character, color, and amount of the drainage. Discard the drainage according to facility policy. Remove gloves. Perform hand hygiene.

—— —— —— 16. Put on clean gloves. If the drain site has a dressing, remove the dressing and assess the site.

—— —— —— 17. Remove gloves and perform hand hygiene.

—— —— —— 18. Cleanse the drain site and redress.

—— —— —— 19. If the drain site is open to air, observe the sutures that secure the drain to the skin. Look for signs of pulling, tearing, swelling, or infection of the surrounding skin. Gently clean the sutures with the gauze pad moistened with normal saline. Dry with a new gauze pad. Apply skin protectant/barrier to the surrounding skin.

—— —— —— 20. Remove and discard gloves. Perform hand hygiene.

—— —— —— 21. Remove all remaining equipment; place the patient in a comfortable position, with side rails up as indicated and bed in the lowest position.

—— —— —— 22. Remove additional PPE, if used. Perform hand hygiene.

—— —— —— 23. Check drain status at least every 4 hours. Empty and reengage suction (compress device) when device is half to two thirds full. Check all wound dressings at least every shift. More frequent checks may be needed if the wound is more complex or dressings become saturated quickly.

Skills Checklist to Accompany Fundamentals of Nursing:
The Art and Science of Person-Centered Care, 9th edition

Name _____ Date _____

Unit _____ Position _____

Instructor/Evaluator: _____ Position _____

SKILL 32-5

Caring for a Hemovac Drain

Goal: The drain is patent and intact.

Columns: Excellent | Satisfactory | Needs Practice | Comments

1. Review the patient's health record for prescribed wound care or the nursing care plan related to wound/drain care. Gather necessary supplies.
2. Perform hand hygiene and put on PPE, if indicated.
3. Identify the patient.
4. Assemble equipment on the overbed table or other surface within reach.
5. Close the curtains around the bed and close the door to the room, if possible. Explain what you are going to do and why you are going to do it to the patient.
6. Assess the patient for possible need for nonpharmacologic pain-reducing interventions or analgesic medication before wound care dressing change. Administer appropriate prescribed analgesic. Allow enough time for analgesic to achieve its effectiveness before beginning the procedure.
7. Place a waste receptacle at a convenient location for use during the procedure.
8. Adjust the bed to a comfortable working height, usually elbow height of the caregiver (VHACEOSH, 2016).
9. Assist the patient to a comfortable position that provides easy access to the drain and/or wound area. Use a bath blanket to cover any exposed area other than the drain. Place a waterproof pad under the drain site.
10. Put on clean gloves; put on mask or face shield, as indicated.
11. Using sterile technique, open a gauze pad, making a sterile field with the outer wrapper.
12. Place the graduated collection container under the drain outlet. ***Without contaminating the outlet, pull off the cap. The chamber will expand completely as it draws in air. Empty the chamber's contents completely into the container. Use the gauze pad to wipe the outlet. Fully compress the chamber by pushing the top and bottom together with your hands. Keep the device tightly compressed while you apply the cap.***

SKILL 32-5

Caring for a Hemovac Drain *(Continued)*

Excellent	Satisfactory	Needs Practice		Comments
——	——	——	13. Device should remain compressed. Check the patency of the equipment. *Make sure the tubing is free from twists and kinks.*	
——	——	——	14. Secure the Hemovac drain to the patient's gown below the wound with a safety pin, *making sure that there is no tension on the tubing.*	
——	——	——	15. Carefully measure and record the character, color, and amount of the drainage. Discard the drainage according to facility policy. Remove gloves. Perform hand hygiene.	
——	——	——	16. Put on clean gloves. If the drain site has a dressing, remove the dressing, assess and clean the site, and replace the dressing. Include cleaning of the sutures with the gauze pad moistened with normal saline. Dry sutures with gauze before applying new dressing.	
——	——	——	17. If the drain site is open to air, observe the sutures that secure the drain to the skin. Look for signs of pulling, tearing, swelling, or infection of the surrounding skin. Gently clean the sutures with the gauze pad moistened with normal saline. Dry with a new gauze pad. Apply skin protectant/barrier to the surrounding skin, if needed.	
——	——	——	18. Remove and discard gloves. Perform hand hygiene.	
——	——	——	19. Remove all remaining equipment; place the patient in a comfortable position, with side rails up as indicated and bed in the lowest position.	
——	——	——	20. Remove additional PPE, if used. Perform hand hygiene.	
——	——	——	21. Check drain status at least every 4 hours. Empty and reengage suction (compress device) when device is half to two thirds full. Check all wound dressings at least every shift. More frequent checks may be needed if the wound is more complex or dressings become saturated quickly.	

Skills Checklist to Accompany Fundamentals of Nursing:
The Art and Science of Person-Centered Care, 9th edition

Name _____ Date _____

Unit _____ Position _____

Instructor/Evaluator: _____ Position _____

SKILL 32-6

Collecting a Wound Culture

Goal: The culture is obtained without evidence of contamination, without exposing the patient to additional pathogens, and without causing discomfort for the patient.

Excellent	Satisfactory	Needs Practice		Comments
___	___	___	1. Review the patient's health record for prescribed orders for obtaining a wound culture. Gather necessary supplies. If possible, obtain the wound culture prior to the start of antimicrobial therapy.	
___	___	___	2. Perform hand hygiene and put on PPE, if indicated.	
___	___	___	3. Identify the patient.	
___	___	___	4. Assemble equipment on the overbed table or other surface within reach.	
___	___	___	5. Close the curtains around the bed and close the door to the room, if possible. Explain to the patient what you are going to do and why you are going to do it.	
___	___	___	6. Assess the patient for possible need for nonpharmacologic pain-reducing interventions or analgesic medication before obtaining the wound culture. Administer appropriate prescribed analgesic. Allow enough time for the analgesic to achieve its effectiveness before beginning the procedure.	
___	___	___	7. Place an appropriate waste receptacle within easy reach for use during the procedure.	
___	___	___	8. Adjust the bed to a comfortable working height, usually elbow height of the caregiver (VHACEOSH, 2016).	
___	___	___	9. Assist the patient to a comfortable position that provides easy access to the wound. If necessary, drape the patient with the bath blanket to expose only the wound area. Place a waterproof pad under the wound site. Check the culture label against the patient's identification bracelet.	
___	___	___	10. If there is a dressing in place on the wound, put on clean gloves and carefully remove the dressing. Note the presence, amount, type, color, and odor of any drainage on the dressings. Place soiled dressings in the appropriate waste receptacle.	
___	___	___	11. Remove gloves and perform hand hygiene.	
___	___	___	12. Assess and clean the wound, ***using a nonantimicrobial cleanser.***	
___	___	___	13. Dry the surrounding skin with gauze dressings. Put on clean gloves.	

SKILL 32-6

Collecting a Wound Culture *(Continued)*

Excellent	Satisfactory	Needs Practice		Comments
—	—	—	14. Twist the cap to loosen the swab on the Culturette tube, or open the separate swab(s) and remove the cap from the culture tube. *Keep the swab and inside of the culture tube(s) sterile.*	
—	—	—	15. If contact with the wound is necessary to separate wound margins to permit insertion of the swab deep into the wound, put a sterile glove on one hand to manipulate the wound margins. Clean gloves may be appropriate for contact with pressure injuries and chronic wounds.	
—	—	—	16. *Identify a 1 cm area of the wound that is free from necrotic tissue.* Carefully insert the swab into this area of clean viable tissue. *Press the swab to apply sufficient pressure to express fluid from the wound tissue and rotate the swab several times. Avoid touching the swab to intact skin at the wound edges.*	
—	—	—	17. Place the swab back in the culture tube. *Do not touch the outside of the tube with the swab.* Secure the cap. Some swab containers have an ampule of medium at the bottom of the tube. It might be necessary to crush this ampule to activate. Follow the manufacturer's instructions for use.	
—	—	—	18. Use another swab if collecting a specimen from another area of the wound or site and repeat the procedure.	
—	—	—	19. Remove gloves and discard them accordingly. Perform hand hygiene.	
—	—	—	20. Put on gloves. Place a dressing on the wound, as appropriate, based on prescribed orders and/or the nursing care plan. Remove gloves. Perform hand hygiene.	
—	—	—	21. After securing the dressing, label dressing with date and time. Remove all remaining equipment; place the patient in a comfortable position, with side rails up as indicated and bed in the lowest position.	
—	—	—	22. Label the specimen according to your institution's guidelines. Information included may include wound site, time the specimen was collected, any antimicrobials the patient is receiving, and the identity of the person who obtained the specimen (Huddleston Cross, 2014). Send or transport specimen to the laboratory in a biohazard bag immediately or within the optimal time from for transport as indicated by facility policy and guidelines.	
—	—	—	23. Remove PPE, if used. Perform hand hygiene.	

Skills Checklist to Accompany Fundamentals of Nursing:
The Art and Science of Person-Centered Care, 9th edition

Name _____ Date _____

Unit _____ Position _____

Instructor/Evaluator: _____ Position _____

Excellent	Satisfactory	Needs Practice	SKILL 32-7 **Applying Negative Pressure Wound Therapy**	Comments
			Goal: The therapy is accomplished without contaminating the wound area, without causing trauma to the wound, and without causing the patient to experience pain or discomfort.	
____	____	____	1. Review the patient's health record for prescribed application of NPWT therapy, including the ordered pressure setting for the device. Gather necessary supplies.	
____	____	____	2. Perform hand hygiene and put on PPE, if indicated.	
____	____	____	3. Identify the patient.	
____	____	____	4. Assemble equipment on the overbed table or other surface within reach.	
____	____	____	5. Close the curtains around the bed and close the door to the room, if possible. Explain what you are going to do and why you are going to do it to the patient.	
____	____	____	6. Assess the patient for possible need for nonpharmacologic pain-reducing interventions or analgesic medication before wound care dressing change. Administer appropriate prescribed analgesic. Allow enough time for the analgesic to achieve its effectiveness before beginning the procedure.	
____	____	____	7. Adjust the bed to a comfortable working height, usually elbow height of the caregiver (VHACEOSH, 2016).	
____	____	____	8. Assist the patient to a comfortable position that provides easy access to the wound area. Position the patient so the cleaning/irrigation solution will flow from the clean end of the wound toward the dirty end. Expose the area and drape the patient with a bath blanket, if needed. Put a waterproof pad under the wound area.	
____	____	____	9. Have the disposal bag or waste receptacle within easy reach for use during the procedure.	
____	____	____	10. Using sterile technique, prepare a sterile field and add all the sterile supplies needed for the procedure to the field. Pour warmed, sterile irrigating solution into the sterile container, as indicated.	
____	____	____	11. Put on a gown, mask, and eye protection.	

Applying Negative Pressure Wound Therapy *(Continued)*

Excellent	Satisfactory	Needs Practice		Comments

Excellent Satisfactory Needs Practice

Comments

12. If NPWT is currently in use, turn off the negative pressure unit. Put on clean, disposable gloves. Loosen the tape on the old dressings by removing in the direction of hair growth and the use of a push–pull method. Push–pull method: lift a corner of the dressing away from the skin, then gently push the skin away from the dressing/adhesive. Continue moving fingers of the opposite hand to support the skin as the product is removed (McNichol et al., 2013). Carefully lift the adhesive from the surrounding skin to prevent medical adhesive–related skin injury (MARSI). Remove the sides/edges first, then the center. If there is resistance, use an adhesive remover (McNichol et al., 2013).

13. Carefully remove the soiled dressings. If any part of the dressing sticks to the underlying skin, use small amounts of sterile saline to help loosen and remove it.

14. Note the presence, amount, type, color, and odor of any drainage on the dressings. *Note the number of pieces of wound contact material removed from the wound. Compare with the documented number from the previous dressing change.*

15. Discard the dressings in the receptacle. Remove your gloves and put them in the receptacle. Perform hand hygiene.

16. Put on sterile gloves. Using sterile technique, clean or irrigate the wound, based on wound care plan and prescribed wound care.

17. Clean the area around the wound with normal saline or prescribed skin cleanser. Dry the surrounding skin with a sterile gauze sponge.

18. Assess the wound for appearance, stage, presence of eschar, granulation tissue, epithelialization, undermining, tunneling, necrosis, sinus tract, and drainage. Assess the appearance of the surrounding tissue. Measure the wound.

19. Remove gloves and perform hand hygiene.

20. Put on sterile gloves. *Wipe intact skin around the wound with a skin protectant/barrier wipe and allow it to dry.*

21. If the use of a wound contact layer (impregnated porous gauze or silicone adhesive contact layer) is indicated, use sterile scissors to cut the wound contact layer to fit the wound bed. Apply wound contact layer to the wound bed.

SKILL 32-7

Applying Negative Pressure Wound Therapy *(Continued)*

Excellent	Satisfactory	Needs Practice		Comments
——	——	——	22. Fit the wound contact material to the shape of the wound. • If using foam wound contact material, use sterile scissors to cut the foam to the shape and measurement of the wound. ***Do not cut foam over the wound.*** More than one piece of foam may be necessary if the first piece is cut too small. Carefully place the foam in the wound. ***Ensure foam-to-foam contact if more than one piece is required.*** • If using gauze wound filler, *carefully place in wound to fill cavity.* • *Note the number of pieces of wound filler placed in the wound.* • *Do not under- or over-fill.*	
——	——	——	23. Trim and place the transparent adhesive drape to cover the wound contact material and an additional 3 to 5 cm border of intact periwound tissue. *Avoid stretching the transparent adhesive drape tight over the wound.*	
——	——	——	24. Choose an appropriate site to apply the connector pad/tubing port. Pinch the transparent adhesive drape and cut a hole through it. Apply the connector pad/tubing port and connective tubing over the hole. Position tubing away from the periwound area and anchor (Schreiber, 2016).	
——	——	——	25. Remove the drainage collection canister from the package and insert into the negative pressure unit until it locks into place. Attach the connective tubing to the canister and check that the clamps on the tubing are open, if present.	
——	——	——	26. Remove gloves and discard. Perform hand hygiene. Turn on the power to the negative pressure unit. Select the prescribed therapy settings (suction and cycle type) and start the device.	
——	——	——	27. *Assess the dressing to ensure seal integrity. The dressing should be collapsed, shrinking to the wound contact material and skin. Observe drainage in tubing.*	
——	——	——	28. Label dressing with date and time. Remove all remaining equipment; place the patient in a comfortable position, with side rails up as indicated and bed in the lowest position.	
——	——	——	29. Remove PPE, if used. Perform hand hygiene.	
——	——	——	30. Check all wound dressings at least every shift. More frequent checks may be needed if the wound is more complex or dressings become saturated quickly. Check negative pressure settings at least every shift. Assess the patient's tolerance of and response to the therapy at least every shift.	

Skills Checklist to Accompany Fundamentals of Nursing:
The Art and Science of Person-Centered Care, 9th edition

Name _____ Date _____

Unit _____ Position _____

Instructor/Evaluator: _____ Position _____

SKILL 32-8

Applying an External Heating Pad

Goal: Desired outcome depends on the patient's nursing diagnosis.

Excellent	Satisfactory	Needs Practice		Comments
____	____	____	1. Review the patient's health record for prescribed order for the application of heat therapy, including frequency, type of therapy, body area to be treated, and length of time for the application. Gather necessary supplies.	
____	____	____	2. Perform hand hygiene and put on PPE, if indicated.	
____	____	____	3. Identify the patient.	
____	____	____	4. Assemble equipment on the overbed table or other surface within reach.	
____	____	____	5. Close the curtains around the bed and close the door to the room if possible. Explain what you are going to do and why you are going to do it to the patient.	
____	____	____	6. Adjust the bed to a comfortable working height, usually elbow height of the caregiver (VHACEOSH, 2016).	
____	____	____	7. Assist the patient to a comfortable position that provides easy access to the area where the heat will be applied; use a bath blanket to cover any other exposed area.	
____	____	____	8. Assess the condition of the skin where the heat is to be applied.	
____	____	____	9. Check that the water in the electronic unit is at the appropriate level. Fill the unit two thirds full or to the fill mark, with distilled water, if necessary. Check the temperature setting on the unit to ensure it is within the safe range.	
____	____	____	10. Attach pad tubing to the electronic unit tubing.	
____	____	____	11. Plug in the unit and warm the pad before use. Apply the aquathermia pad to the prescribed area. Secure with gauze bandage or tape.	
____	____	____	12. Remove PPE, if used, and perform hand hygiene.	
____	____	____	13. *Monitor the condition of the skin and the patient's response to the heat at frequent intervals, according to facility policy. Do not exceed the prescribed length of time for the application of heat.*	

SKILL 32-8

Applying an External Heating Pad *(Continued)*

Excellent	Satisfactory	Needs Practice		Comments
___	___	___	14. After the prescribed time for the treatment (up to 30 minutes), remove the aquathermia pad. ***Do not exceed the prescribed amount of time.*** Reassess the patient and area of application, noting the effect and presence of any adverse effects.	
___	___	___	15. Remove all remaining equipment; place the patient in a comfortable position, with side rails up as indicated and bed in the lowest position.	
___	___	___	16. Remove additional PPE, if used. Perform hand hygiene.	

92

Skills Checklist to Accompany Fundamentals of Nursing:
The Art and Science of Person-Centered Care, 9th edition

Name _____ Date _____

Unit _____ Position _____

Instructor/Evaluator: _____ Position _____

Excellent	Satisfactory	Needs Practice	SKILL 33-1 **Applying and Removing Graduated Compression Stockings**	Comments
			Goal: The stockings are applied and removed with minimal discomfort to the patient.	
___	___	___	1. Review the medical record and medical orders to determine the need for graduated compression stockings.	
___	___	___	2. Perform hand hygiene. Put on PPE, as indicated.	
___	___	___	3. Identify the patient. Explain what you are going to do and the rationale for use of elastic stockings.	
___	___	___	4. Close the curtains around the bed and close the door to the room, if possible.	
___	___	___	5. Adjust the bed to a comfortable working height, usually elbow height of the caregiver (VHACEOSH, 2016).	
___	___	___	6. Assist patient to supine position. If patient has been sitting or walking, have him or her lie down with legs and feet well elevated for at least 15 minutes before applying stockings.	
___	___	___	7. Expose legs one at a time. Wash and dry legs, if necessary. Powder the leg lightly unless patient has a respiratory problem, dry skin, or sensitivity to the powder. If the skin is dry, a lotion may be used. Powders and lotions are not recommended by some manufacturers; check the package material for manufacturer specifications.	
___	___	___	8. Stand at the foot of the bed. Place hand inside stocking and grasp heel area securely. Turn stocking inside-out to the heel area, leaving the foot inside the stocking leg.	
___	___	___	9. With the heel pocket down, ease the stocking foot over the foot and heel. Check that the patient's heel is centered in heel pocket of stocking.	
___	___	___	10. Using your fingers and thumbs, carefully grasp edge of stocking and pull it up smoothly over ankle and calf, toward the knee. Make sure it is distributed evenly.	
___	___	___	11. Pull forward slightly on toe section. If the stocking has a toe window, make sure it is properly positioned. Adjust if necessary to ensure material is smooth.	
___	___	___	12. If the stockings are knee-length, make sure each stocking top is 1 to 2 in below the patella. Make sure the stocking does not roll down.	

Applying and Removing Graduated Compression Stockings *(Continued)*

Excellent	Satisfactory	Needs Practice		Comments
——	——	——	13. If applying thigh-length stocking, continue the application. Flex the patient's leg. Stretch the stocking over the knee.	
——	——	——	14. Pull the stocking over the thigh until the top is 1 to 3 in below the gluteal fold. Adjust the stocking, as necessary, to distribute the fabric evenly. Make sure the stocking does not roll down.	
——	——	——	15. Remove equipment and return patient to a position of comfort. Remove gloves. Raise side rail and lower bed. Place call bell and other essential items within reach.	
——	——	——	16. Remove any other PPE, if used. Perform hand hygiene.	
			Removing Stockings	
——	——	——	17. To remove stocking, grasp top of stocking with your thumb and fingers and smoothly pull stocking off inside-out to heel. Support foot and ease stocking over it.	

Name _____   Date _____

Unit _____   Position _____

Instructor/Evaluator: _____   Position _____

Excellent	Satisfactory	Needs Practice	SKILL 33-2 **Assisting a Patient With Turning in Bed**	Comments
			Goal: The activity takes place without injury to patient or nurse.	
___	___	___	1. Review the medical orders and nursing care plan for patient activity. Identify any movement limitations and the ability of the patient to assist with turning. *Consult patient handling algorithm, if available, to plan appropriate approach to moving the patient.*	
___	___	___	2. Gather any positioning aids or supports, if necessary.	
___	___	___	3. Perform hand hygiene. Put on PPE, as indicated.	
___	___	___	4. Identify the patient. Explain the procedure to the patient.	
___	___	___	5. Close the curtains around the bed and close the door to the room, if possible. Position at least one nurse on either side of the bed. Place pillows, wedges, or any other support to be used for positioning within easy reach. Place the bed at an appropriate and comfortable working height, usually elbow height of the caregiver (VHACEOSH, 2016). Lower both side rails.	
___	___	___	6. If not already in place, position a friction-reducing sheet under the patient.	
___	___	___	7. Using the friction-reducing sheet, move the patient to the edge of the bed, opposite the side to which he or she will be turned. Raise the side rails.	
___	___	___	8. If the patient is able, have the patient grasp the side rail on the side of the bed toward which he or she is turning. Alternately, place the patient's arms across his or her chest and cross his or her far leg over the leg toward which they are turning.	
___	___	___	9. If available, activate the bed-turn mechanism to inflate the side of the bed behind the patient's back.	

SKILL 33-2

Assisting a Patient With Turning in Bed *(Continued)*

Excellent	Satisfactory	Needs Practice		Comments

			10. The nurse on the side of the bed toward which the patient is turning should stand opposite the patient's center with his or her feet spread about shoulder width and with one foot ahead of the other. Tighten your gluteal and abdominal muscles and flex your knees. Use your leg muscles to do the pulling. The other nurse should position his or her hands on the patient's shoulder and hip, assisting to roll the patient to the side. Instruct the patient to pull on the bed rail at the same time. Use the friction-reducing sheet to gently pull the patient over on his or her side.	
			11. Use a pillow or other support behind the patient's back. Pull the shoulder blade forward and out from under the patient.	
			12. Make the patient comfortable and position in proper alignment, using pillows or other supports under the leg and arm, as needed. Readjust the pillow under the patient's head. Elevate the head of the bed as needed for comfort.	
			13. Place the bed in the lowest position, with the side rails up, as indicated. Make sure the call bell and other necessary items are within easy reach.	
			14. Clean transfer aids, per facility policy, if not indicated for single patient use. Remove gloves and other PPE, if used. Perform hand hygiene.	

Skills Checklist to Accompany Fundamentals of Nursing:
The Art and Science of Person-Centered Care, 9th edition

Name _____ Date _____

Unit _____ Position _____

Instructor/Evaluator: _____ Position _____

Excellent	Satisfactory	Needs Practice	SKILL 33-3 **Moving a Patient Up in Bed With the Assistance of Another Caregiver**	Comments
			Goal: The patient remains free from injury and maintains proper body alignment.	
―――	―――	―――	1. Review the medical record and nursing care plan for conditions that may influence the patient's ability to move or to be positioned. Assess for tubes, IV lines, incisions, or equipment that may alter the positioning procedure. Identify any movement limitations. ***Consult patient handling algorithm, if available, to plan appropriate approach to moving the patient.***	
―――	―――	―――	2. Perform hand hygiene and put on PPE, if indicated.	
―――	―――	―――	3. Identify the patient. Explain the procedure to the patient.	
―――	―――	―――	4. Close the curtains around the bed and close the door to the room, if possible. Place the bed at an appropriate and comfortable working height, usually elbow height of the caregiver (VHACEOSH, 2016). Adjust the head of the bed to a flat position or as low as the patient can tolerate. Place the bed in slight Trendelenburg position, if the patient is able to tolerate it.	
―――	―――	―――	5. Remove all pillows from under the patient. Leave one at the head of the bed, leaning upright against the headboard.	
―――	―――	―――	6. Position at least one nurse on either side of the bed, and lower both side rails.	
―――	―――	―――	7. If a friction-reducing sheet (or device) is not in place under the patient, place one under the patient's midsection.	
―――	―――	―――	8. Ask the patient (if able) to bend his or her legs and put his or her feet flat on the bed to assist with the movement.	
―――	―――	―――	9. Have the patient fold the arms across the chest. Have the patient (if able) lift the head with chin on chest.	
―――	―――	―――	10. One nurse should be positioned on each side of the bed, at the patient's midsection, with feet spread shoulder width apart and one foot slightly in front of the other.	
―――	―――	―――	11. If available on bed, engage mechanism to make the bed surface firmer for repositioning.	
―――	―――	―――	12. Grasp the friction-reducing sheet securely, close to the patient's body.	
―――	―――	―――	13. Flex your knees and hips. Tighten your abdominal and gluteal muscles and keep your back straight.	

Moving a Patient Up in Bed With the Assistance of Another Caregiver *(Continued)*

Excellent	Satisfactory	Needs Practice		Comments
___	___	___	14. If possible, the patient can assist with the move by pushing with the legs. Shift your weight back and forth from your back leg to your front leg and count to three. On the count of three, move the patient up in bed. Repeat the process, if necessary, to get the patient to the right position.	
___	___	___	15. Assist the patient to a comfortable position and readjust the pillows and supports, as needed. Take bed out of Trendelenburg position and return bed surface to normal setting, if necessary. Raise the side rails. Place the bed in the lowest position. Make sure the call bell and other necessary items are within easy reach.	
___	___	___	16. Clean transfer aids, per facility policy, if not indicated for single patient use. Remove gloves or other PPE, if used. Perform hand hygiene.	

98

Skills Checklist to Accompany Fundamentals of Nursing:
The Art and Science of Person-Centered Care, 9th edition

Name _____ Date _____

Unit _____ Position _____

Instructor/Evaluator: _____ Position _____

SKILL 33-4

Transferring a Patient From the Bed to a Stretcher

Goal: The patient is transferred without injury to patient or nurse.

Excellent	Satisfactory	Needs Practice		Comments
___	___	___	1. Review the medical record and nursing care plan for any conditions that may influence the patient's ability to move or to be positioned. Assess for tubes, IV lines, incisions, or equipment that may alter the positioning procedure. Identify any movement limitations. ***Consult patient handling algorithm, if available, to plan appropriate approach to moving the patient.***	
___	___	___	2. Perform hand hygiene and put on PPE, if indicated.	
___	___	___	3. Identify the patient. Explain the procedure to the patient.	
___	___	___	4. Close the curtains around the bed and close the door to the room, if possible. Adjust the head of the bed to a flat position or as low as the patient can tolerate. Raise the bed to a height that is even with the transport stretcher (VHACEOSH, 2016). Lower the side rails, if in place.	
___	___	___	5. Place the bath blanket over the patient and remove the top covers from underneath.	
___	___	___	6. If a friction-reducing transfer sheet is not in place under the patient, place one under the patient's midsection. Have patient fold arms against chest and move chin to chest. Use the friction-reducing sheet to move the patient to the side of the bed where the stretcher will be placed. Alternately, place a lateral-assist device under the patient. Follow manufacturer's directions for use.	
___	___	___	7. Position the stretcher next (and parallel) to the bed. ***Lock the wheels on the stretcher and the bed.***	
___	___	___	8. Two nurses should stand on the stretcher side of the bed. A third nurse should stand on the side of the bed without the stretcher.	
___	___	___	9. Use the friction-reducing sheet to roll the patient away from the stretcher. Place the transfer board across the space between the stretcher and the bed, partially under the patient. Roll the patient onto his or her back, so that the patient is partially on the transfer board.	

SKILL 33-4

Transferring a Patient From the
Bed to a Stretcher *(Continued)*

Excellent	Satisfactory	Needs Practice		Comments

10. The nurse on the side of the bed without the stretcher should grasp the friction-reducing sheet at the head and chest areas of the patient. The nurse on the stretcher side of the bed should grasp the friction-reducing sheet at the head and chest, and the other nurse on that side should grasp the friction-reducing sheet at the chest and leg areas of the patient.

11. *At a signal given by one of the nurses, have the nurses standing on the stretcher side of the bed pull the friction-reducing sheet. At the same time, the nurse (or nurses) on the other side push, transferring the patient's weight toward the transfer board, and pushing the patient from the bed to the stretcher.*

12. Once the patient is transferred to the stretcher, remove the transfer board, and secure the patient until the side rails are raised. Raise the side rails. To ensure the patient's comfort, cover the patient with blanket and remove the bath blanket from underneath. Leave the friction-reducing sheet in place for the return transfer. Make sure the call bell and other necessary items are within easy reach.

13. Clean transfer aids, per facility policy, if not indicated for single patient use. Remove gloves and any other PPE, if used. Perform hand hygiene.

Skills Checklist to Accompany Fundamentals of Nursing:
The Art and Science of Person-Centered Care, 9th edition

Name _____   Date _____

Unit _____   Position _____

Instructor/Evaluator: _____   Position _____

Excellent	Satisfactory	Needs Practice	SKILL 33-5 **Transferring a Patient From the Bed to a Chair** **Goal:** The transfer is accomplished without injury to patient or nurse and the patient remains free of any complications of immobility.	Comments
___	___	___	1. Review the medical record and nursing care plan for conditions that may influence the patient's ability to move or to be positioned. Assess for tubes, IV lines, incisions, or equipment that may alter the positioning procedure. Identify any movement limitations. *Consult patient handling algorithm, if available, to plan appropriate approach to moving the patient.*	
___	___	___	2. Perform hand hygiene and put on PPE, as indicated.	
___	___	___	3. Identify the patient. Explain the procedure to the patient.	
___	___	___	4. If needed, move equipment to make room for the chair. Close the curtains around the bed and close the door to the room, if possible.	
___	___	___	5. Place the bed in the lowest position. Raise the head of the bed to a sitting position or as high as the patient can tolerate.	
___	___	___	6. *Make sure the bed brakes are locked. Put the chair next to the bed. If available, lock the brakes of the chair. If the chair does not have brakes, brace the chair against a secure object.*	
___	___	___	7. Encourage the patient to make use of a stand-assist aid, either freestanding or attached to the side of the bed, if available, to move to the side of the bed and to a side-lying position, facing the side of the bed on which the patient will sit.	
___	___	___	8. Lower the side rail, if necessary, and stand near the patient's hips. Stand with your legs shoulder width apart with one foot near the head of the bed, slightly in front of the other foot.	
___	___	___	9. Encourage the patient to make use of the stand-assist device. Assist the patient to sit up on the side of the bed; ask the patient to swing his or her legs over the side of the bed. At the same time, pivot on your back leg to lift the patient's trunk and shoulders. Keep your back straight; avoid twisting.	

Excellent	Satisfactory	Needs Practice		Comments

Excellent	Satisfactory	Needs Practice		
——	——	——	10.	*Stand in front of the patient and assess for any balance problems or complaints of dizziness. Allow the patient's legs to dangle a few minutes before continuing.*
——	——	——	11.	Assist the patient to put on a robe, as necessary, and nonskid footwear.
——	——	——	12.	Wrap the gait belt around the patient's waist, based on assessed need and facility policy.
——	——	——	13.	Stand facing the patient. Spread your feet about shoulder width apart and flex your hips and knees.
——	——	——	14.	Ask the patient to slide his or her buttocks to the edge of the bed until the feet touch the floor. Position yourself as close as possible to the patient, with your foot positioned on the outside of the patient's foot. If a second staff person is assisting, have him or her assume a similar position. Grasp the gait belt.
——	——	——	15.	Encourage the patient to make use of the stand-assist device. If necessary, have second staff person grasp the gait belt on opposite side. Rock back and forth while counting to three. *On the count of three, using the gait belt and your legs (not your back), assist the patient to a standing position.* If indicated, brace your front knee against the patient's weak extremity as he or she stands. Assess the patient's balance and leg strength. If the patient is weak or unsteady, return the patient to bed.
——	——	——	16.	Pivot on your back foot and assist the patient to turn until the patient feels the chair against his or her legs.
——	——	——	17.	Ask the patient to use his arm to steady himself on the arm of the chair while slowly lowering to a sitting position. Continue to brace the patient's knees with your knees and hold the gait belt. Flex your hips and knees when helping the patient sit in the chair.
——	——	——	18.	Assess the patient's alignment in the chair. Remove gait belt, if desired. Depending on patient comfort, it could be left in place to use when returning to bed. Cover with a blanket, if needed. Make sure call bell and other essential items are within easy reach.
——	——	——	19.	Clean transfer aids, per facility policy, if not indicated for single patient use. Remove gloves and any other PPE, if used. Perform hand hygiene.

Skills Checklist to Accompany Fundamentals of Nursing:
The Art and Science of Person-Centered Care, 9th edition

Name _____   Date _____

Unit _____   Position _____

Instructor/Evaluator: _____   Position _____

Excellent	Satisfactory	Needs Practice	SKILL 35-1 **Giving a Back Massage**	Comments
			Goal: The patient reports increased comfort and decreased pain, and is relaxed.	
——	——	——	1. Perform hand hygiene and put on PPE, if indicated.	
——	——	——	2. Identify the patient.	
——	——	——	3. Offer a back massage to the patient and explain the procedure.	
——	——	——	4. Put on gloves, if indicated.	
——	——	——	5. Close the room door and/or the curtain around the bed. Turn down the lights, if possible, and adjust the room temperature for patient comfort (Westman & Blaisdell, 2016).	
——	——	——	6. Assess the patient's pain using an appropriate assessment tool and measurement scale. Ask the patient if he or she has any aversion to touch (Westman & Blaisdell, 2016).	
——	——	——	7. Raise the bed to a comfortable working position, usually elbow height of the caregiver (TVAREF, 2009), and lower the side rail.	
——	——	——	8. Assist the patient to a comfortable position, preferably the prone or side-lying position. Remove the covers and move the patient's gown just enough to expose the patient's back from the shoulders to sacral area. Drape the patient, as needed, with the bath blanket.	
——	——	——	9. Warm the lubricant or lotion in the palm of your hand, or place the container in small basin of warm water. During massage, observe the patient's skin for reddened areas or injury. ***Avoid areas of injury, such as wounds, burns and pressure ulcers and areas with rashes, tubes, and IV lines*** (Westman & Blaisdell, 2016).	
——	——	——	10. Using light, gliding strokes (*effleurage*), apply lotion to patient's shoulders, back, and sacral area.	
——	——	——	11. Place your hands beside each other at the base of the patient's spine and stroke upward to the shoulders and back downward to the buttocks in slow, continuous strokes. Continue for several minutes.	

Giving a Back Massage *(Continued)*

Excellent	Satisfactory	Needs Practice		Comments
——	——	——	12. Massage the patient's shoulders, entire back, areas over iliac crests, and sacrum with circular, stroking motions, keeping hands in contact with the patient's skin. Continue for several minutes, applying additional lotion, as necessary.	
——	——	——	13. Knead the patient's back by gently alternating grasping and compression motions (*pétrissage*).	
——	——	——	14. Complete the massage with additional long, stroking movements that eventually become lighter in pressure.	
——	——	——	15. If excess lotion remains, use the towel to pat the patient dry.	
——	——	——	16. Remove gloves, if worn. Reposition patient's gown and covers. Raise side rail and lower bed. Assist patient to a position of comfort.	
——	——	——	17. Remove additional PPE, if used. Perform hand hygiene.	
——	——	——	18. Evaluate the patient's response to this intervention. Reassess level of discomfort or pain using original assessment tools. Reassess and alter care plan, as appropriate.	

Skills Checklist to Accompany Fundamentals of Nursing:
The Art and Science of Person-Centered Care, 9th edition

Name _____ Date _____

Unit _____ Position _____

Instructor/Evaluator: _____ Position _____

			SKILL 36-1	

SKILL 36-1
Assisting a Patient With Eating

Excellent	Satisfactory	Needs Practice	**Goal:** The patient is able to chew and swallow food.	Comments
⎯	⎯	⎯	1. Check the medical order for the type of diet prescribed for the patient.	
⎯	⎯	⎯	2. Perform hand hygiene and put on PPE, if indicated.	
⎯	⎯	⎯	3. Identify the patient.	
⎯	⎯	⎯	4. Explain the procedure to the patient.	
⎯	⎯	⎯	5. *Assess level of consciousness, for any physical limitations, decreased hearing or visual acuity. If patient uses a hearing aid or wears glasses or dentures, provide, as needed. Ask if the patient has any cultural or religious preferences and food likes and dislikes, if possible.*	
⎯	⎯	⎯	6. Pull the patient's bedside curtain. Assess the abdomen. Ask the patient if he or she has any nausea. Ask the patient if he or she has any difficulty swallowing. Assess the patient for nausea or pain and administer an antiemetic or analgesic, as needed.	
⎯	⎯	⎯	7. Offer to assist the patient with any elimination needs.	
⎯	⎯	⎯	8. Provide hand hygiene and mouth care, as needed.	
⎯	⎯	⎯	9. Remove any bedpans or undesirable equipment and odors, if possible, from the vicinity where the meal will be eaten. Perform hand hygiene.	
⎯	⎯	⎯	10. Open the patient's bedside curtain. Assist to, or position the patient in, a high-Fowler's or sitting position in the bed or chair. Position the bed in the low position if the patient remains in bed.	
⎯	⎯	⎯	11. Place protective covering or towel over the patient if desired and as necessary.	
⎯	⎯	⎯	12. Check food tray to make sure that it is the correct tray before serving. Place tray on the overbed table so the patient can see the food, if able. Ensure that hot foods are hot and cold foods are cold. Use caution with hot beverages, allowing sufficient time for cooling, if needed. Ask the patient for his/her preference related to what foods are desired first. Cut food into small pieces, as needed. Observe swallowing ability throughout the meal.	

SKILL 36-1

Assisting a Patient With Eating *(Continued)*

Excellent	Satisfactory	Needs Practice		Comments
——	——	——	13. If possible, sit facing the patient at the patient's eye level while eating is taking place. If the patient is able, encourage him or her to hold finger foods and feed self as much as possible. Converse with patient during the meal and make eye contact, as appropriate. If, however, the patient has dysphagia, limit questioning or conversation that would require patient response during eating. Play relaxation music if patient desires.	
——	——	——	14. Allow enough time for the patient to chew and swallow the food adequately. The patient may need to rest for short periods during eating.	
——	——	——	15. When the meal is completed or the patient is unable to eat any more, remove the tray from the room. ***Note the amount and types of food consumed. Note the volume of liquid consumed.***	
——	——	——	16. Reposition the overbed table, remove the protective covering, offer hand hygiene, as needed, and offer the bedpan. Assist the patient to a position of comfort and relaxation.	
——	——	——	17. Remove PPE, if used. Perform hand hygiene.	

Skills Checklist to Accompany Fundamentals of Nursing:
The Art and Science of Person-Centered Care, 9th edition

Name _____ Date _____

Unit _____ Position _____

Instructor/Evaluator: _____ Position _____

Excellent	Satisfactory	Needs Practice	SKILL 36-2 **Administering a Tube Feeding**	Comments
			Goal: The patient receives the tube feeding without complaints of nausea or episodes of vomiting.	
——	——	——	1. Gather equipment. Check amount, concentration, type, and frequency of tube feeding in the patient's medical record. Check formula expiration date.	
——	——	——	2. Perform hand hygiene and put on PPE, if indicated.	
——	——	——	3. Identify the patient.	
——	——	——	4. Explain the procedure to the patient. Answer any questions, as needed.	
——	——	——	5. Assemble equipment on overbed table or other surface within reach.	
——	——	——	6. Close the patient's bedside curtain or door. Raise the bed to a comfortable working position, usually elbow height of the caregiver (VHACEOSH, 2016). Perform abdominal assessments as described above.	
——	——	——	7. *Position the patient with HOB elevated at least 30 to 45 degrees or as near normal position for eating as possible.*	
——	——	——	8. Confirm placement of the nasogastric tube in the patient's stomach using at least two methods. The first method utilized should be measurement of the exposed length of tube.	
——	——	——	9. Put on gloves. Unsecure the tube from the patient's gown. Verify the position of the marking on the tube at the nostril. Measure length of exposed tube and compare with the documented length.	
——	——	——	10. Check the pH of and visualize aspirated contents, checking for color and consistency.	
——	——	——	11. If it is not possible to aspirate contents; assessments to check placement are inconclusive; the exposed tube length has changed; or there are any other indications that the tube is not in place, check placement by radiograph (x-ray) of placement of tube, based on facility policy (and ordered by the primary health care provider).	

Administering a Tube Feeding *(Continued)*

Excellent	Satisfactory	Needs Practice		Comments

12. After multiple steps have been taken to ensure that the feeding tube is located in the stomach or small intestine, *aspirate all gastric contents with the syringe and measure to check for gastric residual—the amount of feeding remaining in the stomach.* Return the residual based on facility policy. Proceed with feeding if amount of residual does not exceed facility policy or the limit indicated in the medical record.

13. Flush tube with 30 to 50 mL of water for irrigation. Disconnect syringe from tubing and cap end of tubing while preparing the formula feeding equipment. Remove gloves.

14. Put on gloves before preparing, assembling, and handling any part of the feeding system.

15. Administer feeding.

When Using a Feeding Bag Administration System (Open System)

   a. Label bag and/or tubing with date and time. Hang bag on IV pole and adjust to about 12 in above the stomach. Clamp tubing.

   b. Check the expiration date of the formula. Cleanse top of feeding container with a disinfectant before opening it. Pour formula into feeding bag and allow solution to run through tubing. Close clamp.

   c. Attach feeding administration set to feeding tube, open clamp, and regulate drip according to the medical order, or allow feeding to run in over 30 minutes.

   d. *Add 30 to 60 mL (1 to 2 oz) of water for irrigation to feeding bag when feeding is almost completed and allow it to run through the tube.*

   e. Clamp tubing immediately after water has been instilled. Disconnect feeding administration set from feeding tube. Clamp tube and cover end with cap.

When Using a Large Syringe (Open System)

   a. Remove plunger from 30- or 60-mL syringe.

   b. Attach syringe to feeding tube and pour premeasured amount of tube-feeding formula into syringe. Open the clamp on the feeding tube and allow formula to enter tube. Regulate rate, fast or slow, by height of the syringe. *Do not push formula with syringe plunger.*

SKILL 36-2

Administering a Tube Feeding *(Continued)*

Excellent	Satisfactory	Needs Practice		Comments
—	—	—	c. When feeding is almost completed, *add 30 to 60 mL (1 to 2 oz) of water for irrigation to syringe* and allow it to run through the tube.	
—	—	—	d. When syringe has emptied, hold syringe high, clamp the tube, and disconnect from tube. Cover end with cap.	
			When Using an Enteral Feeding Pump	
—	—	—	a. Close flow-regulator clamp on tubing and fill feeding bag with prescribed formula, as described in Steps 15a and 15b. Amount used depends on facility policy. Place label on container with patient's name, date, and time the feeding was hung.	
—	—	—	b. Hang feeding container on IV pole. Allow solution to flow through tubing.	
—	—	—	c. Connect to feeding pump, following manufacturer's directions. Set rate. Maintain the patient in the upright position throughout the feeding. If the patient needs to lie flat temporarily, pause the feeding. Resume the feeding after the patient's position has been changed back to at least 30 to 45 degrees (Bankhead et al., 2009).	
—	—	—	d. *Check placement of tube and gastric residual every 4 to 6 hours (Bankhead et al., 2009). Flush tube with 30 to 50 mL of water at least every 4 hours during continuous feeding.*	
—	—	—	16. Observe the patient's response during and after tube feeding and assess the abdomen at least once a shift.	
—	—	—	17. *Have patient remain in upright position for at least 1 hour after feeding.*	
—	—	—	18. Remove equipment and return patient to a position of comfort. Remove gloves. Raise side rail and lower bed.	
—	—	—	19. Put on gloves. Wash and clean equipment or replace according to facility policy. Remove gloves.	
—	—	—	20. Remove additional PPE, if used. Perform hand hygiene.	

Skills Checklist to Accompany Fundamentals of Nursing:
The Art and Science of Person-Centered Care, 9th edition

Name _____ Date _____

Unit _____ Position _____

Instructor/Evaluator: _____ Position _____

Excellent	Satisfactory	Needs Practice	SKILL 36-3 **Caring for a Gastrostomy Tube**	Comments
			Goal: The tube is properly positioned with minimal discomfort experienced by the patient.	
——	——	——	1. Gather equipment. Verify the medical order or facility policy and procedure regarding site care.	
——	——	——	2. Perform hand hygiene and put on PPE, if indicated.	
——	——	——	3. Identify the patient.	
——	——	——	4. Explain the procedure to the patient. Answer any questions, as needed.	
——	——	——	5. Assess for presence of pain at the tube-insertion site. If pain is present, offer the patient analgesic medication per the medical order and wait for medication absorption before beginning insertion site care.	
——	——	——	6. Pull the patient's bedside curtain. Assemble equipment on the bedside table, within reach. Raise bed to a comfortable working position, usually elbow height of the caregiver (VHACEOSH, 2016).	
——	——	——	7. Put on gloves. Assess the gastrostomy site, as described above.	
——	——	——	8. Measure the length of exposed tube, comparing it with the initial measurement after insertion. Alternately, examine the mark on the tube at the skin; mark should be at skin level at the insertion site.	
——	——	——	9. For the first 10 days when the gastrostomy tube is new and still has sutures holding it in place, dip a cotton-tipped applicator into sterile saline solution and gently clean around the insertion site, removing any crust or drainage. *Avoid adjusting or lifting the external disk for the first few days after placement, except to clean the area.* After the first 10 days, or when the gastric tube insertion site has healed and the sutures are removed, wet a washcloth and apply a small amount of skin cleanser onto washcloth. Gently cleanse around the insertion, removing any crust or drainage. Rinse site, removing all soap.	
——	——	——	10. Pat skin around insertion site dry.	

Caring for a Gastrostomy Tube *(Continued)*

Excellent	Satisfactory	Needs Practice		Comments
——	——	——	11. If the sutures have been removed, *gently push the tube forward toward the abdomen and rotate the tube. Gently rotate the guard or external bumper 90 degrees at least once a day. Assess that the guard or external bumper is not digging into the surrounding skin. Avoid placing any tension on the tube.*	
——	——	——	12. Leave the site open to air unless there is drainage. If drainage is present, place one thickness of a precut gauze pad or drain sponge under the external bumper and change, as needed, to keep the area dry. Use a skin protectant or barrier cream to prevent skin breakdown.	
——	——	——	13. If the tube is not in use, check that the cap is securely in place.	
——	——	——	14. Assess the integrity of the tape or device used to secure the tube to the stomach.	
——	——	——	15. Remove gloves. Lower the bed and assist the patient to a position of comfort, as needed.	
——	——	——	16. Remove additional PPE, if used. Perform hand hygiene.	

Skills Checklist to Accompany Fundamentals of Nursing:
The Art and Science of Person-Centered Care, 9th edition

Name _____   Date _____

Unit _____   Position _____

Instructor/Evaluator: _____   Position _____

Excellent	Satisfactory	Needs Practice	SKILL 36-4 **Obtaining a Capillary Blood Sample** **for Glucose Testing**	
			Goal: Patient blood glucose levels are accurately monitored.	**Comments**
___	___	___	1. Check the patient's health record or nursing care plan for monitoring schedule. You may decide that additional testing is indicated based on nursing judgment and the patient's condition.	
___	___	___	2. Gather equipment. Check expiration date on blood test strips.	
___	___	___	3. Perform hand hygiene and put on PPE, if indicated.	
___	___	___	4. Identify the patient. Explain the procedure to the patient and instruct the patient about the need for monitoring blood glucose.	
___	___	___	5. Close curtains around the bed and close the door to the room, if possible.	
___	___	___	6. Turn on the monitor.	
___	___	___	7. Enter the patient's identification number or scan his or her identification bracelet, if required, according to facility policy.	
___	___	___	8. Put on nonsterile gloves.	
___	___	___	9. Prepare lancet using aseptic technique.	
___	___	___	10. Remove test strip from the vial. *Recap container immediately.* Test strips also come individually wrapped. *Check that the code number for the strip matches the code number on the monitor screen.*	
___	___	___	11. Insert the strip into the meter according to directions for that specific device. Alternately, strip may be placed in meter after collection of sample on test strip, depending on meter in use.	
___	___	___	12. *Have the patient wash hands with skin cleanser and warm water and dry thoroughly. Alternately, cleanse the skin with an alcohol swab. Allow skin to dry completely.*	
___	___	___	13. Choose a skin site that is intact, warm and free of calluses and edema (Van Leeuwen & Bladh, 2017).	
___	___	___	14. Hold lancet perpendicular to skin and pierce skin with lancet.	

Excellent	Satisfactory	Needs Practice		Comments
			### SKILL 36-4 ## Obtaining a Capillary Blood Sample ## for Glucose Testing *(Continued)*	
——	——	——	15. Encourage bleeding by lowering the hand, making use of gravity. Lightly stroke the finger, if necessary, until a sufficient amount of blood has formed to cover the sample area on the strip, based on monitor requirements (check instructions for monitor). Take care not to squeeze the finger, not to squeeze at puncture site, or not to touch puncture site or blood.	
——	——	——	16. Gently touch a drop of blood to the test strip without smearing it. Depending on meter in use, insert strip into meter after collection of sample on test strip.	
——	——	——	17. Apply pressure to puncture site with a cotton ball or dry gauze. ***Do not use alcohol wipe.***	
——	——	——	18. Read blood glucose results and document the results in EHR or other designated location, based on facility policy. Inform patient of test result.	
——	——	——	19. Turn off meter, remove test strip, and dispose of supplies appropriately. Place lancet in sharps container.	
——	——	——	20. Remove gloves and any other PPE, if used. Perform hand hygiene.	

Skills Checklist to Accompany Fundamentals of Nursing:
The Art and Science of Person-Centered Care, 9th edition

Name _____   Date _____

Unit _____   Position _____

Instructor/Evaluator: _____   Position _____

Excellent	Satisfactory	Needs Practice	SKILL 37-1 **Assessing Bladder Volume Using an Ultrasound Bladder Scanner**	
			Goal: The volume of urine in the bladder is accurately measured.	**Comments**
___	___	___	1. Review the patient's medical record for any limitations in physical activity. Gather equipment.	
___	___	___	2. Perform hand hygiene and put on PPE, if indicated.	
___	___	___	3. Identify the patient.	
___	___	___	4. Close the curtains around the bed and close the door to the room, if possible. Discuss the procedure with the patient and assess the patient's ability to assist with the procedure, as well as personal hygiene preferences.	
___	___	___	5. Adjust the bed to a comfortable working height, usually elbow height of the caregiver (VHACEOSH, 2016). Place the patient in a supine position. Drape the patient. Stand on the patient's right side if you are right-handed, patient's left side if you are left-handed.	
___	___	___	6. Put on clean gloves.	
___	___	___	7. Press the ON button. Wait until the device warms up. Press the SCAN button to turn on the scanning screen.	
___	___	___	8. Press the appropriate biological sex button. The appropriate icon for male or female will appear on the screen.	
___	___	___	9. Clean the scanner head with the appropriate cleaner.	
___	___	___	10. Gently palpate the patient's symphysis pubis (anterior midline junction of pubic bones). Place a generous amount of ultrasound gel or gel pad midline on the patient's abdomen, about 1 to 1.5 in above the symphysis pubis.	
___	___	___	11. Place the scanner head on the gel or gel pad, *with the directional icon on the scanner head toward the patient's head. Aim the scanner head toward the bladder (point the scanner head slightly downward toward the coccyx).* Press and release the scan button	
___	___	___	12. Observe the image on the scanner screen. *Adjust the scanner head to center the bladder image on the crossbars.*	
___	___	___	13. Press and hold the DONE button until it beeps. Read the volume measurement on the screen. Print the results, if required, by pressing PRINT.	

Assessing Bladder Volume Using an Ultrasound Bladder Scanner *(Continued)*

Excellent	Satisfactory	Needs Practice		Comments
——	——	——	14. Use a washcloth or paper towel to remove remaining gel from the patient's skin. Alternately, gently remove gel pad from patient's skin. Return the patient to a comfortable position. Remove your gloves and ensure that the patient is covered.	
——	——	——	15. Lower bed height and adjust the head of the bed to a comfortable position. Reattach call bell, if necessary.	
——	——	——	16. Put on gloves. Clean the scanner head according to the manufacturer's instructions and/or facility policy.	
——	——	——	17. Remove gloves and any additional PPE, if used. Perform hand hygiene.	

Skills Checklist to Accompany Fundamentals of Nursing:
The Art and Science of Person-Centered Care, 9th edition

Name _____ Date _____

Unit _____ Position _____

Instructor/Evaluator: _____ Position _____

Excellent	**Satisfactory**	**Needs Practice**	

SKILL 37-2

Assisting With the Use of a Bedpan

Goal: The patient is able to void with assistance.   **Comments**

Excellent	Satisfactory	Needs Practice	
____	____	____	1. Review the patient's medical record for any limitations in physical activity. Gather equipment.
____	____	____	2. Perform hand hygiene and put on PPE, if indicated.
____	____	____	3. Identify the patient.
____	____	____	4. Assemble equipment on a chair next to the bed within reach.
____	____	____	5. Close curtains around the bed and close the door to the room, if possible. Discuss the procedure with the patient and assess the patient's ability to assist with the procedure, as well as personal hygiene preferences.
____	____	____	6. Unless contraindicated, apply powder to the rim of the bedpan. Place bedpan and cover on a chair next to the bed. Put on gloves.
____	____	____	7. Adjust the bed to a comfortable working height, usually elbow height of the caregiver (VHACEOSH, 2016). Place the patient in a supine position, with the head of the bed elevated about 30 degrees, unless contraindicated.
____	____	____	8. Fold top linen back just enough to allow placement of bedpan. If there is no waterproof pad on the bed and time allows, consider placing a waterproof pad under the patient's buttocks before placing the bedpan.
____	____	____	9. Ask the patient to bend the knees. Have the patient lift his/her hips upward. Assist the patient, if necessary, by placing your hand that is closest to the patient palm up, under the lower back, and assist with lifting. Slip the bedpan into place with the other hand.
____	____	____	10. *Ensure that the bedpan is in proper position and the patient's buttocks are resting on the rounded shelf of the regular bedpan or the shallow rim of the fracture bedpan.*
____	____	____	11. Raise the head of the bed as near to sitting position as tolerated, unless contraindicated. Cover the patient with bed linens.
____	____	____	12. *Place the call bell and toilet tissue within easy reach. Place the bed in the lowest position.* Leave the patient if it is safe to do so. Use side rails appropriately.

Excellent	Satisfactory	Needs Practice		Comments
			SKILL 37-2 ## Assisting With the Use of a Bedpan *(Continued)*	
——	——	——	13. Remove gloves and additional PPE, if used. Perform hand hygiene.	
			Removing the Bedpan	
——	——	——	14. Perform hand hygiene and put on gloves and additional PPE, as indicated. Adjust the bed to a comfortable working height, usually elbow height of the caregiver (VHACEOSH, 2016). Have a receptacle, such as plastic trash bag, handy for discarding tissue.	
——	——	——	15. Lower the head of the bed, if necessary, to about 30 degrees. Remove bedpan in the same manner in which it was offered, being careful to hold it steady. Ask the patient to bend the knees and lift the buttocks up from the bedpan. Assist the patient, if necessary, by placing your hand that is closest to the patient palm up, under the lower back, and assist with lifting. Place the bedpan on the bedside chair and cover it.	
——	——	——	16. If the patient needs assistance with hygiene, wrap tissue around the hand several times, and wipe the patient clean, using one stroke from the pubic area toward the anal area. Discard tissue. Use warm, moist disposable washcloth and skin cleanser to clean the perineal area. Place the patient on his or her side and spread buttocks to clean the anal area.	
——	——	——	17. Do not place toilet tissue in the bedpan if a specimen is required or if output is being recorded. Place toilet tissue in an appropriate receptacle.	
——	——	——	18. Return the patient to a comfortable position. Make sure the linens under the patient are dry. Replace or remove the pad under the patient, as necessary. Remove your gloves and ensure that the patient is covered.	
——	——	——	19. Raise side rail. Lower bed height and adjust the head of the bed to a comfortable position. Reattach call bell.	
——	——	——	20. Offer patient supplies to wash and dry his/her hands, assisting as necessary.	
——	——	——	21. Put on clean gloves. Empty and clean the bedpan, measuring urine in graduated container, as necessary. Discard the trash receptacle with used toilet paper per facility policy.	
——	——	——	22. Remove additional PPE, if used. Perform hand hygiene.	

Skills Checklist to Accompany Fundamentals of Nursing:
The Art and Science of Person-Centered Care, 9th edition

Name _____ Date _____

Unit _____ Position _____

Instructor/Evaluator: _____ Position _____

Excellent	Satisfactory	Needs Practice	SKILL 37-3 **Assisting With the Use of a Urinal**	
			Goal: The patient is able to void with assistance.	**Comments**
——	——	——	1. Review the patient's medical record for any limitations in physical activity. Gather equipment.	
——	——	——	2. Perform hand hygiene and put on PPE, if indicated.	
——	——	——	3. Identify the patient.	
——	——	——	4. Assemble equipment on a chair next to the bed within reach.	
——	——	——	5. Close the curtains around the bed and close the door to the room, if possible. Discuss the procedure with the patient and assess the patient's ability to assist with the procedure, as well as personal hygiene preferences.	
——	——	——	6. Put on gloves.	
——	——	——	7. Assist the patient to an appropriate position, as necessary: standing at the bedside, lying on one side or back, sitting in bed with the head elevated, or sitting on the side of the bed.	
——	——	——	8. If the patient remains in the bed, fold the linens just enough to allow for proper placement of the urinal.	
——	——	——	9. If the patient is not standing, have him spread his legs slightly. *Hold the urinal close to the penis and position the penis completely within the urinal. Keep the bottom of the urinal lower than the penis. If necessary, assist the patient to hold the urinal in place.*	
——	——	——	10. Cover the patient with the bed linens.	
——	——	——	11. Place the call bell and toilet tissue within easy reach. Have a receptacle, such as a plastic trash bag, handy for discarding tissue. Ensure the bed is in the lowest position. Leave patient if it is safe to do so. Use side rails appropriately.	
——	——	——	12. Remove gloves and additional PPE, if used. Perform hand hygiene.	
			Removing the Urinal	
——	——	——	13. Perform hand hygiene. Put on gloves and additional PPE, as indicated.	

Assisting With the Use of a Urinal *(Continued)*

Excellent	Satisfactory	Needs Practice		Comments
——	——	——	14. Pull back the patient's bed linens just enough to remove the urinal. Remove the urinal. Cover the open end of the urinal. Place on the bedside chair. If the patient needs assistance with hygiene, wrap tissue around the hand several times, and wipe the patient dry. Place tissue in a receptacle. Use warm, moist disposable washcloth and skin cleanser to clean perineal area, as necessary, and as per patient request.	
——	——	——	15. Return the patient to a comfortable position. Make sure the linens under the patient are dry. Remove your gloves and ensure that the patient is covered.	
——	——	——	16. Ensure the patient call bell is in reach.	
——	——	——	17. Offer patient supplies to wash and dry his hands, assisting as necessary.	
——	——	——	18. Put on clean gloves. Empty and clean the urinal, measuring urine in a graduated container, as necessary. Discard the trash receptacle with used toilet paper per facility policy.	
——	——	——	19. Remove gloves and additional PPE, if used, and perform hand hygiene.	

Skills Checklist to Accompany Fundamentals of Nursing:
The Art and Science of Person-Centered Care, 9th edition

Name _____   Date _____

Unit _____   Position _____

Instructor/Evaluator: _____   Position _____

Excellent	Satisfactory	Needs Practice	SKILL 37-4 **Applying an External Urinary Sheath (Condom Catheter)**	
			Goal: The patient's urinary elimination is maintained, with a urine output of at least 30 mL/hour, and the bladder is not distended.	**Comments**
___	___	___	1. Gather equipment.	
___	___	___	2. Perform hand hygiene and put on PPE, if indicated.	
___	___	___	3. Identify the patient.	
___	___	___	4. Close the curtains around the bed and close the door to the room, if possible. Discuss the procedure with the patient. Ask the patient if he has any allergies, especially to latex.	
___	___	___	5. Assemble equipment on overbed table or other surface within reach.	
___	___	___	6. Adjust the bed to a comfortable working height, usually elbow height of the caregiver (VHACEOSH, 2016). Stand on the patient's right side if you are right-handed, or on patient's left side if you are left-handed.	
___	___	___	7. Prepare urinary drainage setup or reusable leg bag for attachment to the external urinary sheath.	
___	___	___	8. Position the patient on his back with thighs slightly apart. Drape the patient so that only the area around the penis is exposed. Slide waterproof pad under the patient.	
___	___	___	9. Put on disposable gloves. Trim any long pubic hair that is in contact with the penis.	
___	___	___	10. Clean the genital area with washcloth, skin cleanser, and warm water. If patient is uncircumcised, retract foreskin and clean glans of penis. Replace foreskin. Clean the tip of the penis first, moving the washcloth in a circular motion from the meatus outward. Wash the shaft of the penis using downward strokes toward the pubic area. Rinse and dry. Remove gloves. Perform hand hygiene.	
___	___	___	11. Put on gloves. Apply skin protectant to the penis and allow to dry.	
___	___	___	12. Roll the external urinary sheath outward onto itself. Grasp the penis firmly with the nondominant hand. *Apply the external urinary sheath by rolling it onto the penis with the dominant hand. Leave 1 to 2 in (2.5 to 5 cm) of space between the tip of the penis and the end of the external urinary sheath.*	

Applying an External Urinary Sheath
(Condom Catheter) *(Continued)*

Excellent	Satisfactory	Needs Practice		Comments
——	——	——	13. *Apply pressure to the sheath at the base of the penis for 10 to 15 seconds.*	
——	——	——	14. Connect the external urinary sheath to drainage setup. Avoid kinking or twisting drainage tubing.	
——	——	——	15. Remove gloves. Secure drainage tubing to the patient's inner thigh with Velcro leg strap or tape. Leave some slack in tubing for leg movement.	
——	——	——	16. Assist the patient to a comfortable position. Cover the patient with bed linens. Place the bed in the lowest position.	
——	——	——	17. Secure the drainage bag below the level of the bladder. Check that drainage tubing is not kinked and that movement of side rails does not interfere with the drainage bag.	
——	——	——	18. Remove equipment. Remove gloves and additional PPE, if used. Perform hand hygiene.	

Skills Checklist to Accompany Fundamentals of Nursing:
The Art and Science of Person-Centered Care, 9th edition

Name _____ Date _____

Unit _____ Position _____

Instructor/Evaluator: _____ Position _____

SKILL 37-5

Catheterizing the Female Urinary Bladder

Goal: The patient's urinary elimination is maintained, with a urine output of at least 30 mL/hour, and the patient's bladder is not distended.

Excellent	Satisfactory	Needs Practice		Comments
―	―	―	1. Review the patient's chart for any limitations in physical activity. Confirm the medical order for indwelling catheter insertion.	
―	―	―	2. Gather equipment. Obtain assistance from another staff member, if necessary.	
―	―	―	3. Perform hand hygiene and put on PPE, if indicated.	
―	―	―	4. Identify the patient.	
―	―	―	5. Close the curtains around the bed and close the door to the room, if possible. Discuss the procedure with the patient and assess the patient's ability to assist with the procedure. Ask the patient if she has any allergies, especially to latex or iodine.	
―	―	―	6. Provide good lighting. Artificial light is recommended (use of a flashlight requires an assistant to hold and position it). Place a trash receptacle within easy reach.	
―	―	―	7. Assemble equipment on overbed table or other surface within reach.	
―	―	―	8. Adjust the bed to a comfortable working height, usually elbow height of the caregiver (VHACEOSH, 2016). Stand on the patient's right side if you are right-handed, patient's left side if you are left-handed.	
―	―	―	9. Assist the patient to a dorsal recumbent position with knees flexed, feet about 2 ft apart, with her legs abducted. Drape the patient. Alternately, the Sims', or lateral, position can be used. Place the patient's buttocks near the edge of the bed with her shoulders at the opposite edge and her knees drawn toward her chest. Allow the patient to lie on either side, depending on which position is easiest for the nurse and best for the patient's comfort. Slide waterproof pad under the patient.	
―	―	―	10. Put on clean gloves. Clean the perineal area with washcloth, skin cleanser, and warm water, using a different corner of the washcloth with each stroke. Wipe from above orifice downward toward sacrum (front to back). Rinse and dry. Remove gloves. Perform hand hygiene again.	

Excellent	Satisfactory	Needs Practice		Comments
___	___	___	11. Prepare urine drainage setup if a separate urine collection system is to be used. Secure to bed frame, according to the manufacturer's directions.	
___	___	___	12. Open sterile catheterization tray on a clean overbed table using sterile technique.	
___	___	___	13. Put on sterile gloves. Grasp upper corners of drape and unfold drape without touching nonsterile areas. Fold back a corner on each side to make a cuff over gloved hands. Ask the patient to lift her buttocks and slide sterile drape under her with gloves protected by cuff.	
___	___	___	14. Based on facility policy, position the fenestrated sterile drape. Place a fenestrated sterile drape over the perineal area, exposing the labia. (*Note:* The fenestrated drape is not shown in the remaining illustrations in order to provide a clear view of the procedure.)	
___	___	___	15. Place sterile tray on drape between the patient's thighs.	
___	___	___	16. Open all the supplies. Remove cap from the prefilled sterile saline syringe and attach to the balloon inflation port on the catheter. Open the package of antiseptic swabs. Alternately, fluff cotton balls in a tray before pouring antiseptic solution over them. Open specimen container if specimen is to be obtained.	
___	___	___	17. Lubricate 1 to 2 in of catheter tip.	
___	___	___	18. With thumb and one finger of nondominant hand, spread labia and identify meatus. *Be prepared to maintain separation of labia with one hand until catheter is inserted and urine is flowing well and continuously.* If the patient is in the side-lying position, lift the upper buttock and labia to expose the urinary meatus.	
___	___	___	19. Use the dominant hand to pick up an antiseptic swab or use forceps to pick up a cotton ball. *Clean one labial fold, top to bottom (from above the meatus down toward the rectum), then discard the cotton ball. Using a new cotton ball/swab for each stroke, continue to clean the other labial fold, then directly over the meatus.*	
___	___	___	20. With your noncontaminated, dominant hand, place the drainage end of the catheter in a receptacle. If the catheter is pre-attached to sterile tubing and drainage container (closed drainage system), position the catheter and setup within easy reach on sterile field. Ensure that the clamp on the drainage bag is closed.	

Catheterizing the Female Urinary Bladder *(Continued)*

Excellent	Satisfactory	Needs Practice		Comments
—	—	—	21. *Using your dominant hand, hold the catheter 2 to 3 in from the tip and insert slowly into the urethra. Advance the catheter until there is a return of urine (approximately 2 to 3 in [4.8 to 7.2 cm]). Once urine drains, advance the catheter another 2 to 3 in (4.8 to 7.2 cm). Do not force the catheter through the urethra into the bladder.* Ask the patient to breathe deeply, and rotate the catheter gently if slight resistance is met as the catheter reaches the external sphincter.	
—	—	—	22. Hold the catheter securely at the meatus with your nondominant hand. Use your dominant hand to inflate the catheter balloon. Inject the entire volume of sterile water supplied in a prefilled syringe. Remove the syringe from the port.	
—	—	—	23. Pull gently on the catheter after the balloon is inflated to feel resistance.	
—	—	—	24. Attach the catheter to the drainage system if not already pre-attached.	
—	—	—	25. Remove equipment and dispose of it according to facility policy. Discard syringe in sharps container. Wash and dry the perineal area, as needed.	
—	—	—	26. Remove gloves. *Secure catheter tubing to the patient's inner thigh with a catheter-securing device.* Leave some slack in the catheter for leg movement.	
—	—	—	27. Assist the patient to a comfortable position. Cover the patient with bed linens. Place the bed in the lowest position.	
—	—	—	28. Secure the drainage bag below the level of the bladder. Check that drainage tubing is not kinked and that movement of side rails does not interfere with the catheter or drainage bag.	
—	—	—	29. Put on clean gloves. Obtain urine specimen immediately, if needed, from the drainage bag. Label specimen. Send urine specimen to the laboratory promptly or refrigerate it.	
—	—	—	30. Remove gloves and additional PPE, if used. Perform hand hygiene.	

Skills Checklist to Accompany Fundamentals of Nursing:
The Art and Science of Person-Centered Care, 9th edition

Name _____ Date _____

Unit _____ Position _____

Instructor/Evaluator: _____ Position _____

SKILL 37-6

Catheterizing the Male Urinary Bladder

Goal: The patient's urinary elimination is maintained, with a urine output of at least 30 mL/hour, and the patient's bladder is not distended.

Excellent	Satisfactory	Needs Practice		Comments
___	___	___	1. Review chart for any limitations in physical activity. Confirm the medical order for indwelling catheter insertion.	
___	___	___	2. Gather equipment. Obtain assistance from another staff member, if necessary.	
___	___	___	3. Perform hand hygiene and put on PPE, if indicated.	
___	___	___	4. Identify the patient.	
___	___	___	5. Close the curtains around the bed and close the door to the room, if possible. Discuss the procedure with the patient and assess the patient's ability to assist with the procedure. Ask the patient if he has any allergies, especially to latex or iodine.	
___	___	___	6. Provide good lighting. Artificial light is recommended (use of a flashlight requires an assistant to hold and position it). Place a trash receptacle within easy reach.	
___	___	___	7. Assemble equipment on overbed table or other surface within reach.	
___	___	___	8. Adjust the bed to a comfortable working height, usually elbow height of the caregiver (VHACEOSH, 2016). Stand on the patient's right side if you are right-handed, patient's left side if you are left-handed.	
___	___	___	9. Position the patient on his back with thighs slightly apart. Drape the patient so that only the area around the penis is exposed. Slide waterproof pad under the patient.	
___	___	___	10. Put on clean gloves. Clean the genital area with washcloth, skin cleanser, and warm water. Clean the tip of the penis first, moving the washcloth in a circular motion from the meatus outward. Wash the shaft of the penis using downward strokes toward the pubic area. Rinse and dry. Remove gloves. Perform hand hygiene again.	
___	___	___	11. Prepare urine drainage setup if a separate urine collection system is to be used. Secure to bed frame according to the manufacturer's directions.	
___	___	___	12. Open sterile catheterization tray on a clean overbed table or other flat surface, using sterile technique.	

Excellent	Satisfactory	Needs Practice		Comments
——	——	——	13. Put on sterile gloves. Open sterile drape and place on patient's thighs. Place fenestrated drape with opening over the penis.	
——	——	——	14. Place the catheter setup on or next to the patient's legs on sterile drape.	
——	——	——	15. Open all the supplies. Remove cap from the prefilled sterile saline syringe and attach to the balloon inflation port on the catheter. Open package of antiseptic swabs. Alternately, fluff cotton balls in a tray before pouring antiseptic solution over them. Open specimen container if specimen is to be obtained. Remove cap from syringe prefilled with lubricant.	
——	——	——	16. Place the drainage end of the catheter in a receptacle. If the catheter is preattached to sterile tubing and drainage container (closed drainage system), position catheter and setup within easy reach on sterile field. Ensure that the clamp on drainage bag is closed. Lubricate 1 to 2 in of catheter tip.	
——	——	——	17. Lift the penis with the nondominant hand. Retract the foreskin in an uncircumcised patient. *Be prepared to keep this hand in this position until the catheter is inserted and urine is flowing well and continuously. Use the dominant hand to pick up an antiseptic swab or use forceps to pick up a cotton ball. Using a circular motion, clean the penis, moving from the meatus down the glans of the penis. Repeat this cleansing motion two more times, using a new cotton ball/swab each time. Discard each cotton ball/swab after one use.*	
——	——	——	18. Hold the penis with slight upward tension and perpendicular to the patient's body. Use the dominant hand to pick up the lubricant syringe. *Gently insert the tip of the syringe with a lubricant into the urethra and instill the 10 mL of lubricant.*	
——	——	——	19. Use the dominant hand to pick up the catheter and hold it an inch or two from the tip. Ask the patient to bear down as if voiding. *Insert the catheter tip into the meatus. Ask the patient to take deep breaths. Advance the catheter to the bifurcation or "Y" level of the ports. Do not use force to introduce the catheter.* If the catheter resists entry, ask the patient to breathe deeply and rotate the catheter slightly.	

Excellent	Satisfactory	Needs Practice		Comments

SKILL 37-6
Catheterizing the Male Urinary Bladder *(Continued)*

Excellent	Satisfactory	Needs Practice		Comments
——	——	——	20. Hold the catheter securely at the meatus with your nondominant hand. Use your dominant hand to inflate the catheter balloon. *Inject the entire volume of sterile water supplied in a prefilled syringe. Remove the syringe from the port. Once the balloon is inflated, the catheter may be gently pulled back into place. Replace foreskin, if present, over the catheter.* Lower the penis.	
——	——	——	21. Pull gently on the catheter after the balloon is inflated to feel resistance.	
——	——	——	22. Attach the catheter to drainage system, if necessary.	
——	——	——	23. Remove equipment and dispose of it according to facility policy. Discard syringe in sharps container. Wash and dry the perineal area, as needed.	
——	——	——	24. Remove gloves. Secure catheter tubing to the patient's inner thigh or lower abdomen (with the penis directed toward the patient's chest) with a catheter-securing device or tape. Leave some slack in the catheter for leg movement.	
——	——	——	25. Assist the patient to a comfortable position. Cover the patient with bed linens. Place the bed in the lowest position.	
——	——	——	26. Secure drainage bag below the level of the bladder. Check that drainage tubing is not kinked and that movement of side rails does not interfere with the catheter or drainage bag.	
——	——	——	27. Put on clean gloves. Obtain urine specimen immediately, if needed, from drainage bag. Label specimen. Send urine specimen to the laboratory promptly or refrigerate it.	
——	——	——	28. Remove gloves and additional PPE, if used. Perform hand hygiene.	

Skills Checklist to Accompany Fundamentals of Nursing:
The Art and Science of Person-Centered Care, 9th edition

Name _____   Date _____

Unit _____   Position _____

Instructor/Evaluator: _____   Position _____

Excellent	Satisfactory	Needs Practice	
			SKILL 37-7

Emptying and Changing a Stoma Appliance on a Urinary Diversion

Goal: The stoma appliance is applied correctly to the skin to allow urine to drain freely.

Comments

Excellent	Satisfactory	Needs Practice	
____	____	____	1. Gather equipment.
____	____	____	2. Perform hand hygiene and put on PPE, if indicated.
____	____	____	3. Identify the patient.
____	____	____	4. Close the curtains around the bed and close the door to the room, if possible. Explain what you are going to do and why you are going to do it to the patient. Encourage the patient to observe or participate, if possible.
____	____	____	5. Assemble equipment on overbed table or other surface within reach.
____	____	____	6. Assist the patient to a comfortable sitting or lying position in bed or a standing or sitting position in the bathroom. If the patient is in bed, adjust the bed to a comfortable working height, usually elbow height of the caregiver (VHACEOSH, 2016). Place waterproof pad under the patient at the stoma site.

Emptying the Appliance

Excellent	Satisfactory	Needs Practice	
____	____	____	7. Put on gloves. Hold end of appliance over a bedpan, toilet, or measuring device. Remove the end cap from the spout. Open the spout and empty the contents into the bedpan, toilet, or measuring device.
____	____	____	8. Close the spout. Wipe the spout with toilet tissue. Replace the cap.
____	____	____	9. Remove equipment. Remove gloves. Assist the patient to a comfortable position.
____	____	____	10. If appliance is not to be changed, place bed in lowest position. Remove additional PPE, if used. Perform hand hygiene.

Changing the Appliance

Excellent	Satisfactory	Needs Practice	
____	____	____	11. Place a disposable waterproof pad on the overbed table or other work area. Open the premoistened disposable washcloths or set up the washbasin with warm water and the rest of the supplies. Place a trash bag within reach.

Excellent	Satisfactory	Needs Practice		

Comments

___ ___ ___   12. Put on clean gloves. Place waterproof pad under the patient at the stoma site. Empty the appliance, if necessary, as described in Steps 6 to 8.

___ ___ ___   13. Put on gloves. Gently remove the appliance faceplate, starting at the top and keeping the abdominal skin taut. Remove appliance faceplate from skin by pushing skin from appliance rather than pulling appliance from skin. Apply a silicone-based adhesive remover by spraying or wiping with the remover wipe, as needed.

___ ___ ___   14. Place the appliance in the trash bag, if disposable. If reusable, set aside to wash in lukewarm soap and water and allow to air dry after the new appliance is in place.

___ ___ ___   15. Clean skin around stoma with mild skin cleanser and water or a cleansing agent and a washcloth. Remove all old adhesive from the skin; additional adhesive remover may be used. Do not apply lotion to the peristomal area.

___ ___ ___   16. Gently pat area dry. *Make sure skin around stoma is thoroughly dry.* Assess stoma and condition of surrounding skin.

___ ___ ___   17. Place one or two gauze squares over the stoma opening.

___ ___ ___   18. Apply skin protectant to a 2-in (5-cm) radius around the stoma, and allow it to dry completely, which takes about 30 seconds.

___ ___ ___   19. Lift the gauze squares for a moment and measure the stoma opening, using the measurement guide. Replace the gauze. Trace the same size opening on the back center of the appliance. Cut the opening 1/8 in larger than the stoma size. Use a finger to gently smooth the wafer edges after cutting. Check that the spout is closed and the end cap is in place.

___ ___ ___   20. Remove the paper backing from the appliance faceplate. Quickly remove the gauze squares and discard appropriately; ease the appliance over the stoma. Gently press onto the skin while smoothing over the surface. Apply gentle, even pressure to the appliance for approximately 30 seconds.

___ ___ ___   21. Secure optional belt to appliance and around the patient.

___ ___ ___   22. Remove gloves. Assist the patient to a comfortable position. Cover the patient with bed linens. Place the bed in the lowest position.

___ ___ ___   23. Put on clean gloves. Remove or discard any remaining equipment and assess the patient's response to the procedure.

___ ___ ___   24. Remove gloves and additional PPE, if used. Perform hand hygiene.

Skills Checklist to Accompany Fundamentals of Nursing:
The Art and Science of Person-Centered Care, 9th edition

Name _____   Date _____

Unit _____   Position _____

Instructor/Evaluator: _____   Position _____

SKILL 38-1

Administering a Large-Volume Cleansing Enema

Goal: The patient expels feces and is free from injury with minimal discomfort.

Excellent	Satisfactory	Needs Practice		Comments
____	____	____	1. Verify the order for the enema. Gather equipment.	
____	____	____	2. Perform hand hygiene and put on PPE, if indicated.	
____	____	____	3. Identify the patient.	
____	____	____	4. Explain the procedure to the patient and provide the rationale as to why the enema is needed. Discuss the associated discomforts that may be experienced and possible interventions that may allay this discomfort. Answer any questions, as needed.	
____	____	____	5. Assemble equipment on overbed table or other surface within reach.	
____	____	____	6. Close the curtains around the bed and close the door to the room, if possible. Discuss where the patient will defecate. Have a bedpan, commode, or nearby bathroom ready for use.	
____	____	____	7. Warm the enema solution in the amount ordered, and check the temperature with a thermometer, if available. If a thermometer is not available, warm to room temperature or slightly higher, and test on inner wrist. If tap water is used, adjust the temperature as it flows from the faucet.	
____	____	____	8. Add enema solution to a container. Release clamp and allow fluid to progress through the tube before reclamping.	
____	____	____	9. Adjust the bed to a comfortable working height, usually elbow height of the caregiver (VHACEOSH, 2016). Position the patient on the left side (Sims position), with the upper thigh pulled toward the abdomen, if possible, or the knee–chest position, as dictated by patient comfort and condition. Fold top linen back just enough to allow access to the patient's rectal area. Drape the patient with the bath blanket, as necessary, to maintain privacy and warmth. Place a waterproof pad under the patient's hip.	
____	____	____	10. Put on gloves.	

Excellent	Satisfactory	Needs Practice	SKILL 38-1 **Administering a Large-Volume Cleansing Enema** (*Continued*)
			Comments
—	—	—	11. Elevate solution so that it is no higher than 18 in (45 cm) above level of anus. Plan to give the solution slowly over a period of 5 to 10 minutes. Hang the container on an IV pole or hold it at the proper height.
—	—	—	12. Generously lubricate end of the rectal tube 2 to 3 in (5 to 7 cm). A disposable enema set may have a prelubricated rectal tube.
—	—	—	13. Lift buttock to expose anus. Ask patient to take several deep breaths. Slowly and gently insert the enema tube 3 to 4 in (7 to 10 cm) for an adult. Direct it at an angle pointing toward the umbilicus, not the bladder.
—	—	—	14. If resistance is met while inserting the tube, permit a small amount of solution to enter, withdraw the tube slightly, and then continue to insert it. ***Do not force entry of the tube.*** Ask the patient to take several deep breaths.
—	—	—	15. Introduce solution slowly over a period of 5 to 10 minutes. Hold tubing all the time that solution is being instilled. Assess for dizziness, lightheadedness, nausea, diaphoresis, and clammy skin during administration. ***If the patient experiences any of these symptoms, stop the procedure immediately, monitor the patient's heart rate and blood pressure, and notify the primary care provider.***
—	—	—	16. Clamp tubing or lower container if the patient has the urge to defecate or cramping occurs. Instruct the patient to take small, fast breaths or to pant.
—	—	—	17. After the solution has been given, clamp tubing and remove the tube. Have paper towel ready to receive the tube as it is withdrawn.
—	—	—	18. Return the patient to a comfortable position. Encourage the patient to hold the solution until the urge to defecate is strong, usually in about 5 to 15 minutes. Make sure the linens under the patient are dry. Remove your gloves and ensure that the patient is covered.
—	—	—	19. Raise side rail. Lower bed height and adjust head of bed to a comfortable position.
—	—	—	20. Remove additional PPE, if used. Perform hand hygiene.
—	—	—	21. When patient has a strong urge to defecate, place him or her in a sitting position on a bedpan or assist to a commode or bathroom. Offer toilet tissues, if not in the patient's reach. Stay with the patient or have call bell readily accessible.

SKILL 38-1

Administering a Large-Volume
Cleansing Enema *(Continued)*

Excellent	Satisfactory	Needs Practice		Comments
——	——	——	22. Remind the patient not to flush the commode before you inspect results of enema.	
——	——	——	23. Put on gloves and assist patient, if necessary, with cleaning anal area. Offer washcloths, skin cleanser, and water for handwashing. Remove gloves.	
——	——	——	24. Leave the patient clean and comfortable. Care for equipment properly.	
——	——	——	25. Perform hand hygiene.	

*Skills Checklist to Accompany Fundamentals of Nursing:
The Art and Science of Person-Centered Care, 9th edition*

Name _____ Date _____

Unit _____ Position _____

Instructor/Evaluator: _____ Position _____

Excellent	Satisfactory	Needs Practice	SKILL 38-2 **Inserting a Nasogastric Tube**	Comments
			Goal: The tube is properly inserted and the patient experiences minimal discomfort.	
——	——	——	1. Verify the medical order for insertion of an NG tube. Gather equipment, including selection of the appropriate NG tube.	
——	——	——	2. Perform hand hygiene and put on PPE, if indicated.	
——	——	——	3. Identify the patient.	
——	——	——	4. Explain the procedure to the patient, including the rationale for why the tube is needed. Discuss the associated discomforts that may be experienced and possible interventions that may allay this discomfort. Answer any questions, as needed.	
——	——	——	5. Assemble equipment on overbed table or other surface within reach.	
——	——	——	6. Close the patient's bedside curtain or door. Raise the bed to a comfortable working position, usually elbow height of the caregiver (VHACEOSH, 2016). Assist the patient to high-Fowler's position or elevate the head of the bed 45 degrees if the patient is unable to maintain an upright position. Drape chest with a bath towel or disposable pad. Have emesis basin and tissues within reach.	
——	——	——	7. *Measure the distance to insert the tube by placing the tube tip at the patient's nostril and extending it to the tip of the earlobe and then to tip of the xiphoid process.* Add any extra length based on facility policy. Mark the tube with an indelible marker.	
——	——	——	8. Put on gloves. Lubricate the tip of the tube (at least 2 to 4 in) with water-soluble lubricant. Apply topical anesthetic to the nostril and oropharynx, as appropriate.	
——	——	——	9. After selecting the appropriate nostril, ask the patient to flex the head slightly back against the pillow. Gently insert the tube into the nostril while directing the tube upward and backward along the floor of the nose. The patient may gag when the tube reaches the pharynx. Provide tissues for tearing or watering of eyes. Offer comfort and reassurance to the patient.	

Inserting a Nasogastric Tube *(Continued)*

Excellent	Satisfactory	Needs Practice		Comments

			10. When pharynx is reached, instruct the patient to touch chin to chest. Encourage the patient to sip water through a straw or swallow. Advance the tube in downward and backward direction when patient swallows. Stop when the patient breathes. *If gagging and coughing persist, stop advancing the tube and check placement of the tube with a tongue blade and flashlight.* If the tube is curled, straighten the tube and attempt to advance again. Keep advancing the tube until pen marking is reached. *Do not use force.* Rotate the tube if it meets resistance.	
			11. *Discontinue the procedure and remove the tube if there are signs of distress, such as gasping, coughing, cyanosis, and inability to speak or hum.*	
			12. Secure the tube loosely to the nose or cheek until it is determined that the tube is in the patient's stomach. Confirm placement of the NG tube in the patient's stomach using at least two methods, based on the type of tube in place.	
			a. Obtain radiograph (x-ray) of placement of the tube, based on facility policy and as ordered by the primary care provider.	
			b. Put on gloves. Attach the syringe to end of the tube and aspirate a small amount of stomach contents. If unable to obtain a specimen, reposition the patient and flush the tube with 30 mL of air in a large syringe. Slowly apply negative pressure to withdraw fluid.	
			c. Measure the pH of aspirated fluid using pH paper or a meter. Place a drop of gastric secretions onto pH paper or place small amount in a plastic cup and dip the pH paper into it. Within 30 seconds, compare the color on the paper with the chart supplied by the manufacturer.	
			d. Visualize aspirated contents, checking for color and consistency.	
			e. Measure the length of the exposed tube at the nostril. Mark the tube with an indelible marker.	
			13. After confirmation of the tube placement, secure the tube. Apply skin barrier to the tip and end of the nose and allow to dry. Remove gloves and secure the tube with a commercially prepared device (follow manufacturer's directions) or tape to the patient's nose. To secure with tape:	
			a. Cut a 4-in piece of tape and split bottom 2 in or use packaged nose tape for NG tubes.	

Excellent	Satisfactory	Needs Practice	SKILL 38-2 **Inserting a Nasogastric Tube** *(Continued)*	
				Comments
——	——	——	b. Place unsplit end over the bridge of the patient's nose.	
——	——	——	c. Wrap split ends under and around the NG tube. *Be careful not to pull the tube too tightly against the nose.*	
——	——	——	14. Put on gloves. Clamp the tube and remove the syringe. Cap or attach the tube to suction according to the medical orders. Remove gloves.	
——	——	——	15. Measure the length of the exposed tube. Reinforce marking on the tube at the nostril with indelible ink. Ask the patient to turn his/her head to the side opposite the nostril in which the tube is inserted. Secure the tube to the patient's gown by using rubber band or tape and safety pin. For additional support, tape the tube onto the patient's cheek using a piece of tape. *If a double-lumen tube (e.g., Salem sump) is used, secure the vent above stomach level.* Attach the vent at shoulder level.	
——	——	——	16. Put on gloves. Assist with or provide oral hygiene at 2- to 4-hour intervals. Lubricate the lips generously and clean nares and lubricate, as needed. Offer analgesic throat lozenges or anesthetic spray for throat irritation, if needed.	
——	——	——	17. Remove equipment and return patient to a position of comfort. Remove gloves. Raise side rail and lower bed.	
——	——	——	18. Remove additional PPE, if used. Perform hand hygiene.	

Skills Checklist to Accompany Fundamentals of Nursing:
The Art and Science of Person-Centered Care, 9th edition

Name _____ Date _____

Unit _____ Position _____

Instructor/Evaluator: _____ Position _____

SKILL 38-3

Removing a Nasogastric Tube

Excellent	Satisfactory	Needs Practice	**Goal:** The tube is removed without injury to the patient.	Comments
___	___	___	1. Check medical record for the order for removal of the NG tube.	
___	___	___	2. Perform hand hygiene and put on PPE, if indicated.	
___	___	___	3. Identify the patient.	
___	___	___	4. Explain the procedure to the patient and why this intervention is warranted. Describe that it will entail a quick few moments of discomfort. Perform key abdominal assessments as described above.	
___	___	___	5. Pull the patient's bedside curtain. Raise the bed to a comfortable working position; usually elbow height of the caregiver (VHACEOSH, 2016). Assist the patient to a 30- to 45-degree position. Place a towel or disposable pad across the patient's chest. Give tissues and emesis basin to the patient.	
___	___	___	6. Put on gloves. Discontinue suction and separate the tube from suction. Detach the tube from the patient's gown and carefully remove adhesive tape from the patient's nose.	
___	___	___	7. Check placement and *flush with 10 mL of water or normal saline solution (optional) or clear with 30 to 50 mL of air.*	
___	___	___	8. Clamp the tube with fingers by doubling the tube on itself. *Instruct the patient to take a deep breath and hold it. Quickly and carefully remove the tube while the patient holds breath.* Coil the tube in the disposable pad as you remove it from the patient.	
___	___	___	9. Dispose of the tube per facility policy. Remove gloves. Perform hand hygiene.	
___	___	___	10. Offer mouth care to the patient and facial tissue to blow nose. Lower the bed and assist the patient to a position of comfort, as needed.	
___	___	___	11. Remove equipment and raise side rail and lower bed.	

Removing a Nasogastric Tube *(Continued)*

Excellent	Satisfactory	Needs Practice		Comments
⎯	⎯	⎯	12. Put on gloves and measure the amount of NG drainage in the collection device. Record the measurement on the output flow record, subtracting irrigant fluids if necessary. Add solidifying agent to NG drainage and dispose of drainage according to facility policy.	
⎯	⎯	⎯	13. Remove additional PPE, if used. Perform hand hygiene.	

Skills Checklist to Accompany Fundamentals of Nursing:
The Art and Science of Person-Centered Care, 9th edition

Name _____ Date _____

Unit _____ Position _____

Instructor/Evaluator: _____ Position _____

Excellent	Satisfactory	Needs Practice	SKILL 38-4 **Irrigating a Nasogastric Tube Connected to Suction**	
			Goal: The tube maintains patency with irrigation and the patient remains free from injury.	**Comments**
___	___	___	1. Gather equipment. Verify the medical order or facility policy and procedure regarding frequency of irrigation, solution type, and amount of irrigant. Check expiration dates on irrigating solution and irrigation set.	
___	___	___	2. Perform hand hygiene and put on PPE, if indicated.	
___	___	___	3. Identify the patient.	
___	___	___	4. Explain the procedure to the patient and why this intervention is needed. Answer any questions, as needed. Perform key abdominal assessments as described above.	
___	___	___	5. Assemble equipment on overbed table or other surface within reach.	
___	___	___	6. Pull the patient's bedside curtain. Raise bed to a comfortable working position, usually elbow height of the caregiver (VHACEOSH, 2016). Assist the patient to 30- to 45-degree position, unless this is contraindicated. Pour the irrigating solution into container.	
___	___	___	7. Put on gloves. Place waterproof pad on the patient's chest, under connection of the NG tube and suction tubing. ***Check placement of the NG tube.***	
___	___	___	8. Draw up 30 mL of irrigation solution (or amount indicated in the order or policy) into the syringe.	
___	___	___	9. Clamp the NG tube near connection site. Disconnect the tube from the suction apparatus and lay on a disposable pad or towel, or hold both tubes upright in nondominant hand.	
___	___	___	10. Place tip of the syringe in the tube. ***If Salem sump or double-lumen tube is used, make sure that the syringe tip is placed in the drainage port and not in blue air vent.*** Hold the syringe upright and gently insert the irrigant (or allow solution to flow in by gravity if facility policy or medical order indicates). ***Do not force solution into the tube.***	

Excellent

Satisfactory

Needs Practice

Irrigating a Nasogastric Tube
Connected to Suction *(Continued)*

Comments

—— —— —— 11. *If unable to irrigate the tube, reposition patient and attempt irrigation again. Inject 10 to 20 mL of air and aspirate again. If repeated attempts to irrigate the tube fail, consult with primary care provider or follow facility policy.*

—— —— —— 12. After irrigant has been instilled, hold the end of the NG tube over irrigation tray or emesis basin. Observe for return flow of NG drainage into an available container. Alternately, you may reconnect the NG tube to suction and observe the return drainage as it drains into the suction container.

—— —— —— 13. If not already done, reconnect drainage port to suction, if ordered.

—— —— —— 14. Inject air into blue air vent after irrigation is complete. Position the blue air vent above the patient's stomach.

—— —— —— 15. Remove gloves. Lower the bed and raise side rails, as necessary. Assist the patient to a position of comfort. Perform hand hygiene.

—— —— —— 16. Put on gloves. Measure returned solution, if collected outside of suction apparatus. Rinse equipment if it will be reused. Label with the date, patient's name, room number, and purpose (for NG tube/irrigation).

—— —— —— 17. Remove gloves and additional PPE, if used. Perform hand hygiene.

Skills Checklist to Accompany Fundamentals of Nursing:
The Art and Science of Person-Centered Care, 9th edition

Name _____ Date _____

Unit _____ Position _____

Instructor/Evaluator: _____ Position _____

Excellent	Satisfactory	Needs Practice	SKILL 38-5 **Emptying and Changing an Ostomy Appliance**	Comments
			Goal: The stoma appliance is applied correctly to the skin to allow stool to drain freely.	
___	___	___	1. Gather equipment.	
___	___	___	2. Perform hand hygiene and put on PPE, if indicated.	
___	___	___	3. Identify the patient.	
___	___	___	4. Close the curtains around the bed and close the door to the room, if possible. Explain what you are going to do and why you are going to do it to the patient. Encourage the patient to observe or participate, if possible.	
___	___	___	5. Assemble equipment on overbed table or other surface within reach.	
___	___	___	6. Assist the patient to a comfortable sitting or lying position in bed or a standing or sitting position in the bathroom. If the patient is in bed, adjust the bed to a comfortable working height, usually elbow height of the caregiver (VHACEOSH, 2016). Place waterproof pad under the patient at the stoma site.	

Emptying an Appliance

___	___	___	7. Put on gloves. Remove clamp and fold end of appliance or pouch upward like a cuff.	
___	___	___	8. Empty contents into bedpan, toilet, or measuring device.	
___	___	___	9. Wipe the lower 2 in of the appliance or pouch with toilet tissue or paper towel.	
___	___	___	10. Uncuff edge of appliance or pouch and apply clip or clamp, or secure Velcro closure. Ensure the curve of the clamp follows the curve of the patient's body. Remove gloves. Assist the patient to a comfortable position.	
___	___	___	11. If appliance is not to be changed, place bed in lowest position. Remove additional PPE, if used. Perform hand hygiene.	

Changing an Appliance

___	___	___	12. Place a disposable pad on the work surface. Open the pre-moistened disposable washcloths or set up the washbasin with warm water and the rest of the supplies. Place a trash bag within reach.	

Excellent	Satisfactory	Needs Practice		Comments

Emptying and Changing an Ostomy Appliance *(Continued)*

Excellent	Satisfactory	Needs Practice	
——	——	——	13. Put on clean gloves. Place waterproof pad under the patient at the stoma site. Empty the appliance as described in Steps 7–10.
——	——	——	14. Put on gloves. Start at the top of the appliance and keep the abdominal skin taut. Gently remove pouch faceplate from skin by pushing skin from the appliance rather than pulling the appliance from skin. Apply a silicone-based adhesive remover by spraying or wiping with the remover wipe.
——	——	——	15. Place the appliance in the trash bag, if disposable. If reusable, set aside to wash in lukewarm soap and water and allow to air dry after the new appliance is in place.
——	——	——	16. Use toilet tissue to remove any excess stool from the stoma. Cover the stoma with gauze pad. Clean the skin around the stoma with skin cleanser and water or a cleansing agent and a washcloth. Remove all old adhesive from the skin; use an adhesive remover, as necessary. Do not apply lotion to the peristomal area.
——	——	——	17. Gently pat area dry. ***Make sure the skin around the stoma is thoroughly dry.*** Assess the stoma and the condition of the surrounding skin.
——	——	——	18. Apply skin protectant to a 2-in (5-cm) radius around the stoma, and allow it to dry completely, which takes about 30 seconds.
——	——	——	19. Lift the gauze squares for a moment and measure the stoma opening, using the measurement guide. Replace the gauze. Trace the same-size opening on the back center of the appliance. Cut the opening 1/8 in larger than the stoma size. Using a finger, gently smooth the wafer edges after cutting.
——	——	——	20. Remove the paper backing from the appliance faceplate. Quickly remove the gauze squares and ease the appliance over the stoma. Gently press onto the skin while smoothing over the surface. Apply gentle, even pressure to the appliance for approximately 30 seconds.
——	——	——	21. Close the bottom of the appliance or pouch by folding the end upward and using the clamp or clip that comes with the product, or secure the Velcro closure. Ensure the curve of the clamp follows the curve of the patient's body.

Emptying and Changing an
Ostomy Appliance *(Continued)*

Excellent **Satisfactory** **Needs Practice**

Comments

___ ___ ___ 22. Remove gloves. Assist the patient to a comfortable position. Cover the patient with bed linens. Place the bed in the lowest position.

___ ___ ___ 23. Put on clean gloves. Remove or discard equipment and assess the patient's response to the procedure.

___ ___ ___ 24. Remove gloves and additional PPE, if used. Perform hand hygiene.

Skills Checklist to Accompany Fundamentals of Nursing:
The Art and Science of Person-Centered Care, 9th edition

Name _____ Date _____

Unit _____ Position _____

Instructor/Evaluator: _____ Position _____

SKILL 39-1

Using a Pulse Oximeter

Goal: The patient exhibits arterial blood oxygen saturation within acceptable parameters, or greater than 95%.

Excellent	Satisfactory	Needs Practice		Comments
___	___	___	1. Review health record for any health problems that would affect the patient's oxygenation status. Gather equipment.	
___	___	___	2. Perform hand hygiene and put on PPE, if indicated.	
___	___	___	3. Identify the patient.	
___	___	___	4. Assemble equipment to the bedside stand or overbed table or other surface within reach.	
___	___	___	5. Close the curtains around the bed and close the door to the room, if possible. Explain what you are going to do and why you are going to do it to the patient.	
___	___	___	6. Select an appropriate site for application of the sensor.	
___	___	___	a. Use the patient's index, middle, or ring finger.	
___	___	___	b. Check the proximal pulse and capillary refill closest to the site.	
___	___	___	c. If circulation to the site is inadequate, consider using the earlobe, forehead, or bridge of the nose. Use the appropriate oximetry sensor for the chosen site.	
___	___	___	d. Use a toe only if lower extremity circulation is not compromised.	
___	___	___	7. Select proper equipment:	
___	___	___	a. If one finger is too large for the probe, use a smaller finger.	
___	___	___	b. Use probes appropriate for the patient's age and size. Use a pediatric probe for a small adult, if necessary.	
___	___	___	c. Check if the patient is allergic to adhesive. A nonadhesive finger clip or reflectance sensor is available.	
___	___	___	8. Prepare the monitoring site. Cleanse the selected area with the alcohol wipe or disposable cleansing cloth, as necessary. Allow the area to dry. If necessary, remove the nail polish and artificial nails after checking pulse oximeter's manufacturer's instructions.	
___	___	___	9. Attach the probe securely to the skin. *Make sure that the light-emitting sensor and the light-receiving sensor are aligned opposite each other (not necessary to check if placed on the forehead or bridge of the nose).*	

Using a Pulse Oximeter *(Continued)*

Excellent	Satisfactory	Needs Practice		Comments
——	——	——	10. Connect the sensor probe to the pulse oximeter, turn the oximeter on, and check operation of the equipment (audible beep, fluctuation of the bar of light or waveform on the face of the oximeter).	
——	——	——	11. Set alarms on the pulse oximeter. Check the manufacturer's alarm limits for high and low pulse rate settings.	
——	——	——	12. Check oxygen saturation at regular intervals, as ordered by the primary care provider, nursing assessment, and signaled by alarms. Monitor the hemoglobin level.	
——	——	——	13. Remove the sensor on a regular basis and check for skin irritation or signs of pressure (every 2 hours for spring-tension sensor or every 4 hours for adhesive finger or toe sensor).	
——	——	——	14. Clean nondisposable sensors according to the manufacturer's directions. Remove PPE, if used. Perform hand hygiene.	

Skills Checklist to Accompany Fundamentals of Nursing:
The Art and Science of Person-Centered Care, 9th edition

Name _____ Date _____

Unit _____ Position _____

Instructor/Evaluator: _____ Position _____

Excellent	Satisfactory	Needs Practice	SKILL 39-2 **Suctioning the Oropharyngeal and Nasopharyngeal Airways**	Comments
			Goal: The patient exhibits improved breath sounds and a clear, patent airway.	
——	——	——	1. Gather equipment.	
——	——	——	2. Perform hand hygiene and put on PPE, if indicated.	
——	——	——	3. Identify the patient.	
——	——	——	4. Assemble equipment on the overbed table or other surface within reach.	
——	——	——	5. Close the curtains around the bed and close the door to the room, if possible.	
——	——	——	6. Determine the need for suctioning. Verify the suction order in the patient's medical record, if necessary. *Assess for pain or the potential to cause pain. Administer pain medication, as prescribed, before suctioning.*	
——	——	——	7. Explain what you are going to do and the reason for suctioning to the patient, even if the patient does not appear to be alert. Reassure the patient you will interrupt the procedure if he or she indicates respiratory difficulty.	
——	——	——	8. Adjust the bed to a comfortable working height, usually elbow height of the caregiver (VHACEOSH, 2016). Lower the side rail closest to you. *If conscious, place the patient in a semi-Fowler's position. If unconscious, place the patient in the lateral position, facing you.* Move the bedside table close to your work area and raise it to waist height.	
——	——	——	9. Place towel or waterproof pad across the patient's chest.	
——	——	——	10. *Adjust suction to appropriate pressure.*	
——	——	——	• Using a wall unit for adults and adolescents: no more than 150 mm Hg; neonates: no more than 80 mm Hg; infants: no more than 100 mm Hg; children: no more than 125 mm Hg (Hess et al., 2016).	
——	——	——	• For a portable unit for an adult: 10 to 15 cm Hg; neonates: 6 to 8 cm Hg; infants: 8 to 10 cm Hg; children: 8 to 10 cm Hg; adolescents: 8 to 15 cm Hg.	
——	——	——	*Put on a disposable, clean glove and occlude the end of the connecting tubing to check suction pressure.* Place the connecting tubing in a convenient location.	

Suctioning the Oropharyngeal and Nasopharyngeal Airways (Continued)

Excellent	Satisfactory	Needs Practice		Comments

___ ___ ___	11. Open sterile suction package using aseptic technique. The open wrapper or container becomes a sterile field to hold other supplies. Carefully remove the sterile container, touching only the outside surface. Set it up on the work surface and pour sterile saline into it.	
___ ___ ___	12. Place a small amount of water-soluble lubricant on the sterile field, taking care to avoid touching the sterile field with the lubricant package.	
___ ___ ___	13. Increase the patient's supplemental oxygen level or apply supplemental oxygen per facility policy or primary care provider order.	
___ ___ ___	14. Put on face shield or goggles and mask. Put on sterile gloves. *The dominant hand will manipulate the catheter and must remain sterile. The nondominant hand is considered clean rather than sterile and will control the suction valve (Y-port) on the catheter.* In the home setting and other community-based settings, maintenance of sterility is not necessary.	
___ ___ ___	15. With the dominant gloved hand, pick up the sterile catheter. Pick up the connecting tubing with the nondominant hand and connect the tubing and suction catheter.	
___ ___ ___	16. Moisten the catheter by dipping it into the container of sterile saline. Occlude Y-tube to check suction.	
___ ___ ___	17. Encourage the patient to take several deep breaths.	
___ ___ ___	18. Apply lubricant to the first 2 to 3 in of the catheter, using the lubricant that was placed on the sterile field.	
___ ___ ___	19. Remove the oxygen delivery device, if appropriate. Do not apply suction as the catheter is inserted. Hold the catheter between your thumb and forefinger.	
___ ___ ___	20. Insert the catheter:	
___ ___ ___	a. **For nasopharyngeal suctioning,** gently insert the catheter through the naris and along the floor of the nostril toward the trachea. Roll the catheter between your fingers to help advance it. Advance the catheter approximately 5 to 6 in to reach the pharynx.	
___ ___ ___	b. **For oropharyngeal suctioning,** insert catheter through the mouth, along the side of the mouth toward the trachea. Advance the catheter 3 to 4 in to reach the pharynx.	

Suctioning the Oropharyngeal and Nasopharyngeal Airways *(Continued)*

Excellent	Satisfactory	Needs Practice		Comments
——	——	——	21. *Apply suction by intermittently occluding the Y-port on the catheter with the thumb of your nondominant hand and gently rotating the catheter as it is being withdrawn. Do not suction for more than 10 to 15 seconds at a time.*	
——	——	——	22. Replace the oxygen delivery device using your nondominant hand, if appropriate, and have the patient take several deep breaths.	
——	——	——	23. Flush the catheter with saline. Assess the effectiveness of suctioning and repeat, as needed, and according to the patient's tolerance. Wrap the suction catheter around your dominant hand between attempts.	
——	——	——	24. *Allow at least a 30-second to 1-minute interval if additional suctioning is needed. No more than three suction passes should be made per suctioning episode. Alternate the naris, unless contraindicated, if repeated suctioning is required.* Do not force the catheter through the naris. Encourage the patient to cough and deep breathe between suctioning. *Suction the oropharynx after suctioning the nasopharynx.*	
——	——	——	25. When suctioning is completed, remove gloves from the dominant hand over the coiled catheter, pulling them off inside out. Remove the glove from the nondominant hand and dispose of gloves, catheter, and container with solution in the appropriate receptacle. Assist the patient to a comfortable position. Raise bed rail and place bed in the lowest position.	
——	——	——	26. Turn off suction. Remove supplemental oxygen placed for suctioning, if appropriate. Remove face shield or goggles and mask. Perform hand hygiene.	
——	——	——	27. Perform oral hygiene after suctioning.	
——	——	——	28. Reassess the patient's respiratory status, including respiratory rate, effort, oxygen saturation, and lung sounds.	
——	——	——	29. Remove additional PPE, if used. Perform hand hygiene.	

Skills Checklist to Accompany Fundamentals of Nursing:
The Art and Science of Person-Centered Care, 9th edition

Name _____ Date _____

Unit _____ Position _____

Instructor/Evaluator: _____ Position _____

Excellent	Satisfactory	Needs Practice	SKILL 39-3 — **Administering Oxygen by Nasal Cannula**	Comments
			Goal: The patient exhibits an oxygen saturation level within acceptable parameters.	
____	____	____	1. Review the medical order to verify the use of the nasal cannula, flow rate, and administration parameters. Gather equipment.	
____	____	____	2. Perform hand hygiene and put on PPE, if indicated.	
____	____	____	3. Identify the patient.	
____	____	____	4. Assemble equipment on the overbed table or other surface within reach.	
____	____	____	5. Close the curtains around the bed and close the door to the room, if possible.	
____	____	____	6. Explain what you are going to do and the reason for doing it to the patient. Review safety precautions necessary when oxygen is in use.	
____	____	____	7. Connect the nasal cannula to the oxygen source, with humidification, if appropriate. Adjust the flow rate as ordered. Check that oxygen is flowing out of prongs.	
____	____	____	8. Place prongs in the patient's nostrils. Place tubing over and behind each ear with adjuster comfortably under chin. Alternatively, the tubing may be placed around the patient's head, with the adjuster at the back or base of the head. Place gauze pads at ear beneath the tubing or commercially available ear pads, as necessary.	
____	____	____	9. Adjust the fit of the cannula, as necessary. Tubing should be snug but not tight against the skin.	
____	____	____	10. *Encourage patients to breathe through the nose, with the mouth closed.*	
____	____	____	11. Reassess the patient's respiratory status, including the respiratory rate, effort, and lung sounds. Note any signs of respiratory distress, such as tachypnea, nasal flaring, use of accessory muscles, or dyspnea.	
____	____	____	12. Remove PPE, if used. Perform hand hygiene.	
____	____	____	13. Put on clean gloves. Remove and clean the cannula and assess nares at least every 8 hours, or according to facility recommendations. Check nares for evidence of irritation or bleeding.	

148

Skills Checklist to Accompany Fundamentals of Nursing:
The Art and Science of Person-Centered Care, 9th edition

Name _____   Date _____

Unit _____   Position _____

Instructor/Evaluator: _____   Position _____

			SKILL 39-4	
Excellent	**Satisfactory**	**Needs Practice**	**Administering Oxygen by Mask**	
			Goal: The patient exhibits an oxygen saturation level within acceptable parameters.	**Comments**
⎯ ⎯ ⎯			1. Review the medical order to verify the use of the particular mask, flow rate/concentration, and administration parameters. Gather equipment.	
⎯ ⎯ ⎯			2. Perform hand hygiene and put on PPE, if indicated.	
⎯ ⎯ ⎯			3. Identify the patient.	
⎯ ⎯ ⎯			4. Assemble equipment on the overbed table or other surface within reach.	
⎯ ⎯ ⎯			5. Close the curtains around the bed and close the door to the room, if possible.	
⎯ ⎯ ⎯			6. Explain what you are going to do and the reason for doing it to the patient. Review safety precautions necessary when oxygen is in use.	
⎯ ⎯ ⎯			7. Attach the face mask to the oxygen source (with humidification, if appropriate, for the specific mask). Start the flow of oxygen at the specified rate. For a mask with a reservoir, be sure to allow oxygen to fill the bag before proceeding to the next step.	
⎯ ⎯ ⎯			8. Position face mask over the patient's nose and mouth. *Adjust the elastic strap so that the mask fits snugly but comfortably on the face.* Adjust to the prescribed flow rate.	
⎯ ⎯ ⎯			9. If the patient reports irritation or you note redness, use gauze pads under the elastic strap at pressure points to reduce irritation to ears and scalp.	
⎯ ⎯ ⎯			10. Reassess the patient's respiratory status, including respiratory rate, effort, and lung sounds. Note any signs of respiratory distress, such as tachypnea, nasal flaring, use of accessory muscles, or dyspnea.	
⎯ ⎯ ⎯			11. Remove PPE, if used. Perform hand hygiene.	
⎯ ⎯ ⎯			12. *Remove the mask and dry the skin every 2 to 3 hours if the oxygen is running continuously. Do not use powder around the mask.*	

Skills Checklist to Accompany Fundamentals of Nursing:
The Art and Science of Person-Centered Care, 9th edition

Name _____ Date _____

Unit _____ Position _____

Instructor/Evaluator: _____ Position _____

Excellent	Satisfactory	Needs Practice	SKILL 39-5 **Providing Care of a Tracheostomy Tube**	
			Goal: The patient exhibits a tracheostomy tube and site free from drainage, secretions, and skin irritation or breakdown.	**Comments**
⎯⎯	⎯⎯	⎯⎯	1. Gather equipment.	
⎯⎯	⎯⎯	⎯⎯	2. Perform hand hygiene and put on PPE, if indicated.	
⎯⎯	⎯⎯	⎯⎯	3. Identify the patient.	
⎯⎯	⎯⎯	⎯⎯	4. Assemble equipment on the overbed table or other surface within reach.	
⎯⎯	⎯⎯	⎯⎯	5. Close the curtains around the bed and close the door to the room, if possible.	
⎯⎯	⎯⎯	⎯⎯	6. Determine the need for tracheostomy care. *Assess the patient's pain and administer pain medication, if indicated.*	
⎯⎯	⎯⎯	⎯⎯	7. Explain what you are going to do and the reason for doing it to the patient, even if the patient does not appear to be alert. Reassure the patient you will interrupt the procedure if he or she indicates respiratory difficulty.	
⎯⎯	⎯⎯	⎯⎯	8. Adjust the bed to a comfortable working position, usually elbow height of the caregiver (VHACEOSH, 2016). Lower the side rail closest to you. *If conscious, place the patient in a semi-Fowler's position. If unconscious, place the patient in the lateral position, facing you.* Move the overbed table close to your work area and raise it to waist height. Place a trash receptacle within easy reach of the work area.	
⎯⎯	⎯⎯	⎯⎯	9. Put on face shield or goggles and mask. Suction tracheostomy, if necessary. If tracheostomy has just been suctioned, remove soiled site dressing and discard before removal of gloves used to perform suctioning.	
			Cleaning the Tracheostomy: Disposable Inner Cannula	
⎯⎯	⎯⎯	⎯⎯	10. Carefully open the package with the new disposable inner cannula, taking care not to contaminate the cannula or the inside of the package. Carefully open the package with the sterile cotton-tipped applicators, taking care not to contaminate them. Open the sterile cup or basin and fill 0.5 in deep with saline. Open the plastic disposable bag and place within reach on work surface.	

Providing Care of a Tracheostomy Tube *(Continued)*

Excellent	Satisfactory	Needs Practice		Comments
——	——	——	11. Put on disposable gloves.	
——	——	——	12. Remove the oxygen source if one is present. Stabilize the outer cannula and faceplate of the tracheostomy with your nondominant hand. Grasp the locking mechanism of the inner cannula with your dominant hand. Press the tabs and release the lock. Gently remove the inner cannula and place in disposal bag. If not already removed, remove site dressing and dispose of it in the trash.	
——	——	——	13. Working quickly, discard gloves and put on sterile gloves. Pick up the new inner cannula with your dominant hand; stabilize the faceplate with your nondominant hand and gently insert the new inner cannula into the outer cannula. Press the tabs to allow the lock to grab the outer cannula. Reapply oxygen source, if needed.	
			Applying Clean Dressing and Holder	
——	——	——	14. Remove oxygen source, if necessary. Dip cotton-tipped applicator or gauze sponge in cup or basin with sterile saline and clean stoma under faceplate. Use each applicator or sponge only once, moving from stoma site outward.	
——	——	——	15. Pat skin gently with dry 4 × 4 gauze sponge.	
——	——	——	16. Slide commercially prepared tracheostomy dressing or prefolded non–cotton-filled 4 × 4-in dressing under the faceplate.	
——	——	——	17. Change the tracheostomy holder:	
——	——	——	a. *Obtain the assistance of a second person to hold the tracheostomy tube in place while the old collar is removed and the new collar is placed.*	
——	——	——	b. Open the package for the new tracheostomy collar.	
——	——	——	c. Both nurses should put on clean gloves.	
——	——	——	d. One nurse holds the faceplate while the other pulls up the Velcro tabs. Gently remove the collar.	
——	——	——	e. The first nurse continues to hold the tracheostomy faceplate.	
——	——	——	f. The other nurse places the collar around the patient's neck and inserts first one tab, then the other, into the openings on the faceplate and secures the Velcro tabs on the tracheostomy holder.	
——	——	——	g. Check the fit of the tracheostomy collar. You should be able to fit one finger between the neck and the collar. Check to make sure that the patient can flex the neck comfortably. Reapply the oxygen source, if necessary.	

Excellent	Satisfactory	Needs Practice		Comments

Providing Care of a Tracheostomy Tube *(Continued)*

Excellent	Satisfactory	Needs Practice		
___	___	___	18. Remove gloves. Remove face shield or goggles and mask. Assist the patient to a comfortable position. Raise the bed rail and place the bed in the lowest position.	
___	___	___	19. Reassess the patient's respiratory status, including respiratory rate, effort, oxygen saturation, and lung sounds.	
___	___	___	20. Remove additional PPE, if used. Perform hand hygiene.	

Skills Checklist to Accompany Fundamentals of Nursing:
The Art and Science of Person-Centered Care, 9th edition

Name _____ Date _____

Unit _____ Position _____

Instructor/Evaluator: _____ Position _____

Excellent	Satisfactory	Needs Practice	SKILL 39-6 **Suctioning a Tracheostomy: Open System**	Comments
			Goal: The patient exhibits improved breath sounds and a clear, patent airway.	
——	——	——	1. Gather equipment.	
——	——	——	2. Perform hand hygiene and put on PPE, if indicated.	
——	——	——	3. Identify the patient.	
——	——	——	4. Assemble equipment on the overbed table or other surface within reach.	
——	——	——	5. Close the curtains around the bed and close the door to the room, if possible.	
——	——	——	6. Determine the need for suctioning. Verify the suction order in the patient's medical record. *Assess for pain or the potential to cause pain. Administer pain medication, as prescribed, before suctioning.*	
——	——	——	7. Explain to the patient what you are going to do and the reason for doing it, even if the patient does not appear to be alert. Reassure the patient you will interrupt the procedure if he or she indicates respiratory difficulty.	
——	——	——	8. Adjust the bed to a comfortable working position, usually elbow height of the caregiver (VHACEOSH, 2016). Lower the side rail closest to you. *If conscious, place the patient in a semi-Fowler's position. If unconscious, place the patient in the lateral position, facing you.*	
——	——	——	9. Place a towel or waterproof pad across the patient's chest.	
——	——	——	10. *Adjust suction to appropriate pressure.*	
——	——	——	• Using a wall unit for adults and adolescents: no more than 150 mm Hg; neonates: no more than 80 mm Hg; infants: no more than 100 mm Hg; children: no more than 125 mm Hg (Hess et al., 2016).	
——	——	——	• For a portable unit for an adult: 10 to 15 cm Hg; neonates: 6 to 8 cm Hg; infants: 8 to 10 cm Hg; children: 8 to 10 cm Hg; adolescents: 8 to 15 cm Hg. Put on a disposable, clean glove and occlude the end of the connecting tubing to check suction pressure. Place the connecting tubing in a convenient location. If using, place the resuscitation bag connected to oxygen within convenient reach.	

SKILL 39-6
Suctioning a Tracheostomy:
Open System (Continued)

Excellent	Satisfactory	Needs Practice		Comments
——	——	——	11. Open the sterile suction package using aseptic technique. The open wrapper or container becomes a sterile field to hold other supplies. Carefully remove the sterile container, touching only the outside surface. Set it up on the work surface and pour sterile saline into it.	
——	——	——	12. Put on face shield or goggles and mask. Put on sterile gloves. *The dominant hand will manipulate the catheter and must remain sterile. The nondominant hand is considered clean rather than sterile and will control the suction valve (Y-port) on the catheter.*	
——	——	——	13. With the dominant gloved hand, pick up the sterile catheter. Pick up the connecting tubing with the nondominant hand and connect the tubing and suction catheter.	
——	——	——	14. Moisten the catheter by dipping it into the container of sterile saline, unless it is a silicone catheter. Occlude Y-tube to check suction.	
——	——	——	15. Using your nondominant hand and a manual resuscitation bag, hyperventilate the patient, delivering three to six breaths or use the sigh mechanism on a mechanical ventilator.	
——	——	——	16. Remove the manual resuscitation bag or open the adapter on the mechanical ventilator tubing with your nondominant hand.	
——	——	——	17. Using your dominant hand, gently and quickly insert the catheter into the trachea. *Advance the catheter to the predetermined length. Do not occlude the Y-port when inserting the catheter.*	
——	——	——	18. Apply suction by intermittently occluding the Y-port on the catheter with the thumb of your nondominant hand, and gently rotate the catheter as it is being withdrawn. *Do not suction for more than 10 to 15 seconds at a time.*	
——	——	——	19. Hyperventilate the patient using your nondominant hand and a manual resuscitation bag, delivering three to six breaths. Replace the oxygen delivery device, if applicable, using your nondominant hand and have the patient take several deep breaths. If the patient is mechanically ventilated, close the adapter on the mechanical ventilator tubing and use the sigh mechanism on a mechanical ventilator.	
——	——	——	20. Flush the catheter with saline. Assess the effectiveness of suctioning and repeat, as needed, according to the patient's tolerance. Wrap the suction catheter around your dominant hand between attempts.	

Suctioning a Tracheostomy: Open System *(Continued)*

Excellent	Satisfactory	Needs Practice		Comments
——	——	——	21. *Allow at least a 30-second to 1-minute interval if additional suctioning is needed. Do not make more than three suction passes per suctioning episode. Encourage the patient to cough and deep breathe between suctioning attempts.* Suction the oropharynx after suctioning the trachea. Do not reinsert in the tracheostomy after suctioning the mouth.	
——	——	——	22. Perform oral hygiene after tracheal suctioning.	
——	——	——	23. When suctioning is completed, coil the catheter in one hand. Remove the glove from the hand over the coiled catheter (catheter remains inside glove), pulling the glove off inside out. Remove the glove from the other hand, pulling inside out, and dispose of gloves, catheter, and container with solution in the appropriate receptacle. Assist the patient to a comfortable position. Raise the bed rail and place the bed in the lowest position.	
——	——	——	24. Turn off suction. Remove supplemental oxygen placed for suctioning, if appropriate. Remove face shield or goggles and mask. Perform hand hygiene.	
——	——	——	25. Reassess the patient's respiratory status, including respiratory rate, effort, oxygen saturation, and lung sounds.	
——	——	——	26. Remove additional PPE, if used. Perform hand hygiene.	

Skills Checklist to Accompany Fundamentals of Nursing:
The Art and Science of Person-Centered Care, 9th edition

Name _____ Date _____

Unit _____ Position _____

Instructor/Evaluator: _____ Position _____

Excellent	Satisfactory	Needs Practice	SKILL 40-1 **Initiating a Peripheral Venous Access IV Infusion** **Goal:** The access device is inserted on the first attempt, using sterile technique.	Comments
___	___	___	1. Verify the IV solution order on the eMAR/MAR with the medical order. Consider the appropriateness of the prescribed therapy in relation to the patient. Clarify any inconsistencies. Check the patient's chart for allergies. Check solution for color, leaking, and expiration date. Know techniques for IV insertion, precautions, and purpose of the IV solution administration, if ordered. Gather necessary supplies.	
___	___	___	2. Perform hand hygiene and put on PPE, if indicated.	
___	___	___	3. Identify the patient.	
___	___	___	4. Assemble equipment to the bedside stand or overbed table or other surface within reach.	
___	___	___	5. Close the curtains around the bed and close the door to the room, if possible. Explain what you are going to do and why you are going to do it to the patient. Ask the patient about allergies to medications, tape, or skin antiseptics, as appropriate. If considering using a local anesthetic, inquire about allergies for these substances as well.	
___	___	___	6. If using a local anesthetic, explain the rationale and procedure to the patient. Apply the anesthetic to a few potential insertion sites. Allow sufficient time for the anesthetic to take effect.	
			Prepare the IV Solution and Administration Set	
___	___	___	7. Compare the IV container label with the eMAR/MAR. Remove IV bag from outer wrapper, if indicated. Check expiration dates. Scan bar code on container, if necessary. Compare patient identification band with the eMAR/MAR. Alternately, label the solution container with the patient's name, solution type, additives, date, and time. Complete a time strip for the infusion and apply to IV container.	
___	___	___	8. Maintain aseptic technique when opening sterile packages and IV solution. Remove administration set from the package. Apply label to the tubing reflecting the day/date for next set change, per facility guidelines.	

Initiating a Peripheral Venous Access
IV Infusion (Continued)

Excellent	Satisfactory	Needs Practice		Comments
—	—	—	9. Close the roller clamp or slide the clamp on the IV administration set. Invert the IV solution container and remove the cap on the entry site, taking care not to touch the exposed entry site. Remove the cap from the spike on the administration set. Using a twisting and pushing motion, insert the administration set spike into the entry site of the IV container. Alternately, follow the manufacturer's directions for insertion	
—	—	—	10. Hang the IV container on the IV pole. Squeeze the drip chamber and fill at least halfway.	
—	—	—	11. Open the IV tubing clamp, and allow fluid to move through the tubing. Follow the additional manufacturer's instructions for specific electronic infusion pump, as indicated. ***Allow fluid to flow until all air bubbles have disappeared and the entire length of the tubing is primed (filled) with IV solution.*** Close the clamp. Alternately, some brands of tubing may require removal of the cap at the end of the IV tubing to allow fluid to flow. Maintain its sterility. After fluid has filled the tubing, recap the end of the tubing.	
—	—	—	12. If an electronic device is to be used, follow the manufacturer's instructions for inserting the tubing into the device.	
			Initiate Peripheral Venous Access	
—	—	—	13. Place the patient in low-Fowler's position in bed. Place a protective towel or pad under the patient's arm.	
—	—	—	14. Provide emotional support, as needed.	
—	—	—	15. Open the short extension tubing package. Attach the needleless connector or end cap, if not in place. Clean the needleless connector or end cap with alcohol wipe. Insert a syringe with normal saline into the extension tubing. Fill the extension tubing with normal saline and place the extension tubing and syringe back on the package, within easy reach.	
—	—	—	16. Select and palpate for an appropriate vein.	
—	—	—	17. If the site is hairy and facility policy permits, clip a 2-in area around the intended entry site.	
—	—	—	18. Put on gloves.	
—	—	—	19. Apply a tourniquet 3 to 4 in above the venipuncture site to obstruct venous blood flow and distend the vein. Direct the ends of the tourniquet away from the entry site. Make sure the radial pulse is still present.	

Excellent	Satisfactory	Needs Practice	

Comments

____ ____ ____ 20. Instruct the patient to hold the arm lower than the heart.

____ ____ ____ 21. Ask the patient to open and close the fist. Observe and palpate for a suitable vein. Try the following techniques if a vein cannot be felt:

____ ____ ____   a. Lightly stroke the vein downward.

____ ____ ____   b. Remove tourniquet and place warm, dry compresses over intended vein for 10 to 15 minutes.

____ ____ ____ 22. *Cleanse the site with >5% chlorhexidine, or according to facility policy. Press the applicator against the skin and apply chlorhexidine using a gentle back and forth motion. Do not wipe or blot. Allow to dry completely for at least 30 seconds (INS, 2016a).*

____ ____ ____ 23. Using the nondominant hand placed about 1 or 2 in below the entry site, hold the skin taut against the vein. *Avoid touching the prepared site.* Ask the patient to remain still while performing the venipuncture.

____ ____ ____ 24. Align the IV catheter on top of the vein; enter the skin gently, holding the catheter by the hub in your dominant hand, bevel side up, at a 10- to 15-degree angle. Insert the catheter from directly over the vein or from the side of the vein. While following the course of the vein, advance the needle or catheter into the vein. A sensation of "give" can be felt when the needle enters the vein.

____ ____ ____ 25. Continue to hold the skin taut. When blood returns through the catheter and/or the flashback chamber of the catheter, use the push-off tab to separate the catheter from the needle stylet and advance the catheter into the vein until the hub is at the venipuncture site. The exact technique depends on the type of device used.

____ ____ ____ 26. Release the tourniquet. Activate the safety mechanism on the needle stylet. Compress the skin well above the catheter tip to stop the flow of blood. Quickly remove the protective cap from the extension tubing and attach it to the catheter hub and tighten the Luer lock. Stabilize the catheter or needle with your nondominant hand.

____ ____ ____ 27. Continue to stabilize the catheter or needle and pull back on the syringe to assess for blood return, then, flush gently with the saline, observing the site for infiltration and leaking. Remove the syringe from the end cap.

Excellent	Satisfactory	Needs Practice		Comments

			28. Open the skin protectant wipe. Apply the skin protectant to the site, making sure to apply—at minimum—the area to be covered with the dressing. Place a sterile transparent dressing and/or catheter securing/stabilization device over the venipuncture site. Loop the tubing near the entry site, and anchor with tape (nonallergenic) close to the site.	
			29. Label the IV dressing with the date, time, site, and type and size of the catheter placed.	
			30. Using an antimicrobial swab, vigorously scrub the needleless connector or end cap on the extension tubing and allow to dry. Remove the end cap from the administration set. Insert the end of the administration set into the needleless connector or end cap. Loop the administration set tubing near the entry site, and anchor with tape (nonallergenic) close to the site. Remove gloves.	
			31. Open the clamp on the administration set. Set the flow rate and begin the fluid infusion. Alternately, start the flow of solution by releasing the clamp on the tubing and counting the drops. Adjust until the correct drop rate is achieved. Assess the flow of the solution and function of the infusion device. Inspect the insertion site for signs of infiltration.	
			32. Apply an IV securement/stabilization device if not already in place as part of the dressing, as indicated, based on facility policy. Explain to the patient the purpose of the device and the importance of safeguarding the site when using the extremity.	
			33. Apply a passive disinfection cap to each access site on the administration set. Using an antimicrobial swab, vigorously scrub each access site cap on the administration set tubing and allow to dry. Attach a passive disinfection cap to each site.	
			34. Remove equipment and return the patient to a position of comfort. Lower the bed, if not in the lowest position.	
			35. Remove additional PPE, if used. Perform hand hygiene.	
			36. Return to check the flow rate and observe the IV site for infiltration and/or other complications 30 minutes after starting infusion, and at least hourly thereafter. Ask the patient if he/she is experiencing any pain or discomfort related to the IV infusion.	

Skills Checklist to Accompany Fundamentals of Nursing:
The Art and Science of Person-Centered Care, 9th edition

Name _____ Date _____

Unit _____ Position _____

Instructor/Evaluator: _____ Position _____

SKILL 40-2

Monitoring an IV Site and Infusion

Excellent	Satisfactory	Needs Practice		Comments
			Goal: The patient remains free from complications and demonstrates signs and symptoms of fluid balance.	
——	——	——	1. Verify IV solution order on the eMAR/MAR with the medical order. Consider the appropriateness of the prescribed therapy in relation to the patient. Clarify any inconsistencies. Check the patient's medical record for allergies. Check for color, leaking, and expiration date. Know the purpose of the IV administration.	
——	——	——	2. *Monitor IV infusion every hour or per facility policy. More frequent checks may be necessary if medication is being infused.*	
——	——	——	3. Perform hand hygiene and put on PPE, if indicated.	
——	——	——	4. Identify the patient.	
——	——	——	5. Close the curtains around the bed and close the door to the room, if possible. Explain what you are going to do and why you are doing it to the patient.	
——	——	——	6. If an electronic infusion device is being used, check settings, alarm, and indicator lights. Check set infusion rate. Note position of fluid in IV container in relation to time tape. Teach the patient about the alarm features on the electronic infusion device.	
——	——	——	7. If IV is infusing via gravity, check the drip chamber and time the drops.	
——	——	——	8. Check the tubing for anything that might interfere with the flow. Be sure clamps are in the open position.	
——	——	——	9. Observe the dressing for leakage of IV solution.	
——	——	——	10. Inspect the site for swelling, leakage at the site, coolness, or pallor, which may indicate infiltration. Ask if the patient is experiencing any pain or discomfort. If any of these symptoms are present, the IV will need to be removed and restarted at another site. Check facility policy for treating infiltration.	

SKILL 40-2
Monitoring an IV Site and Infusion *(Continued)*

Excellent	Satisfactory	Needs Practice		Comments

—— —— —— 11. Inspect the site for redness, swelling, and heat. Palpate for induration. Ask if the patient is experiencing pain. These findings may indicate phlebitis, making it necessary to discontinue and restart the IV at another site. Grade phlebitis. Check facility policy for treatment of phlebitis. Notify the primary health care provider for severe (Grade 3 or 4) phlebitis (INS, 2016a).

—— —— —— 12. Check for local manifestations (redness, pus, warmth, induration, and pain) that may indicate an infection is present at the site. Also check for systemic manifestations (chills, fever, tachycardia, hypotension) that may accompany local infection at the site. If signs of infection are present, discontinue the IV and notify the primary care provider. Be careful not to disconnect the IV tubing when putting on patient's hospital gown or assisting the patient with movement.

—— —— —— 13. Be alert for additional complications of IV therapy, such as fluid overload or bleeding.

—— —— —— a. Fluid overload can result in signs of cardiac and/or respiratory failure. Monitor intake and output and vital signs. Assess for edema and auscultate lung sounds. Ask if the patient is experiencing any shortness of breath.

—— —— —— b. Check for bleeding at the site.

—— —— —— 14. If appropriate, instruct the patient to call for assistance if any discomfort is noted at the site, solution container is nearly empty, flow has changed in any way, or if the electronic pump alarm sounds.

—— —— —— 15. Remove PPE, if used. Perform hand hygiene.

Skills Checklist to Accompany Fundamentals of Nursing:
The Art and Science of Person-Centered Care, 9th edition

Name _____   Date _____

Unit _____   Position _____

Instructor/Evaluator: _____   Position _____

Excellent	Satisfactory	Needs Practice	SKILL 40-3 **Changing a Peripheral Venous Access Site Dressing** **Goal:** The patient exhibits an access site that is clean, dry, and without evidence of any signs and symptoms of infection, infiltration, or phlebitis. In addition, the dressing will be clean, dry, and intact and the patient will not experience injury.	Comments
____	____	____	1. Determine the need for a dressing change. Check facility policy. Gather equipment.	
____	____	____	2. Perform hand hygiene and put on PPE, if indicated.	
____	____	____	3. Identify the patient.	
____	____	____	4. Assemble equipment to the bedside stand or overbed table or other surface within reach.	
____	____	____	5. Close the curtains around the bed and close the door to the room, if possible. Explain what you are going to do and why you are going to do it to the patient. Ask the patient about allergies to tape and skin antiseptics.	
____	____	____	6. Put on gloves. Place a towel or disposable pad under the arm with the venous access. If the solution is currently infusing, temporarily stop the infusion. Hold the catheter in place with your nondominant hand. Beginning at the device hub, *gently pull the dressing perpendicular to the skin toward the insertion site, carefully removing the old dressing and/or stabilization/securing device.* Avoid inadvertently dislodging the catheter, as it may be adhered to the dressing (INS, 2016a). Use adhesive remover as necessary. Discard the dressing.	
____	____	____	7. *Inspect the IV site for the presence of phlebitis (inflammation), infection, or infiltration.* If noted, discontinue and relocate IV.	
____	____	____	8. *Cleanse the site with an antiseptic solution, such as chlorhexidine, or according to facility policy. Press the applicator against the skin and apply chlorhexidine using a gentle back and forth motion. Do not wipe or blot. Allow to dry completely for at least 30 seconds (INS, 2016a).*	
____	____	____	9. Open the skin protectant wipe. Apply it to the site, making sure to cover at minimum the area to be covered with the dressing. Allow to dry. Place the sterile transparent dressing and/or catheter securing/stabilization device over the venipuncture site.	

Changing a Peripheral Venous Access
Site Dressing *(Continued)*

Excellent	Satisfactory	Needs Practice		Comments
——	——	——	10. Label the dressing with date, time of change, and initials. Loop the tubing near the entry site, and anchor with tape (nonallergenic) close to the site. Resume fluid infusion, if indicated. Check that IV flow is accurate and system is patent.	
——	——	——	11. Apply an IV securement/stabilization device if not already in place as part of the dressing, as indicated, based on facility policy. Explain to the patient the purpose of the device and the importance of safeguarding the site when using the extremity.	
——	——	——	12. Remove equipment. Ensure the patient's comfort. Remove gloves. Lower the bed, if not in the lowest position.	
——	——	——	13. Remove additional PPE, if used. Perform hand hygiene.	

Skills Checklist to Accompany Fundamentals of Nursing:
The Art and Science of Person-Centered Care, 9th edition

Name _____   Date _____

Unit _____   Position _____

Instructor/Evaluator: _____   Position _____

Excellent	Satisfactory	Needs Practice	SKILL 40-4 **Capping for Intermittent Use and Flushing a Peripheral Venous Access Device** **Goal:** The patient remains free of injury and any signs and symptoms of IV complications.	Comments
____	____	____	1. Determine the need for conversion to an intermittent access. Verify medical order. Check facility policy. Gather equipment.	
____	____	____	2. Perform hand hygiene and put on PPE, if indicated.	
____	____	____	3. Identify the patient.	
____	____	____	4. Assemble equipment to the bedside stand or overbed table or other surface within reach.	
____	____	____	5. Close the curtains around the bed and close the door to the room, if possible. Explain what you are going to do and why you are going to do it to the patient. Ask the patient about allergies to tape and skin antiseptics.	
____	____	____	6. Assess the IV site.	
____	____	____	7. If using an electronic infusion device, stop the device. Close the roller clamp on the administration set. If using gravity infusion, close the roller clamp on the administration set.	
____	____	____	8. Put on gloves. Close the clamp on the short extension tubing connected to the IV catheter in the patient's arm.	
____	____	____	9. Remove the administration set tubing from the needleless connector or end cap on the extension set. Using an antimicrobial swab, vigorously scrub the needleless connector or end cap on the extension tubing and allow to dry.	
____	____	____	10. Insert the saline flush syringe into the needleless connector or end cap on the extension tubing. Pull back on the syringe to aspirate the catheter for positive blood return. If positive, instill the solution over 1 minute or flush the line according to facility policy. Remove the syringe and reclamp the extension tubing.	
____	____	____	11. If necessary, loop the extension tubing near the entry site and anchor it with tape (nonallergenic) close to the site.	
____	____	____	12. Using an antimicrobial swab, vigorously scrub the needleless connector or end cap on the extension tubing and allow to dry. Attach a passive disinfection cap.	
____	____	____	13. Remove equipment. Ensure the patient's comfort. Remove gloves. Lower the bed, if not in the lowest position.	
____	____	____	14. Remove additional PPE, if used. Perform hand hygiene.	

Skills Checklist to Accompany Fundamentals of Nursing:
The Art and Science of Person-Centered Care, 9th edition

Name _____ Date _____

Unit _____ Position _____

Instructor/Evaluator: _____ Position _____

Excellent	Satisfactory	Needs Practice	SKILL 40-5 **Administering a Blood Transfusion**	Comments
			Goal: The patient receives the blood transfusion without any evidence of a transfusion reaction or complication.	
___	___	___	1. Verify the medical order for transfusion of a blood product. Verify the completion of informed consent documentation in the medical record. Verify any medical order for pretransfusion medication. If ordered, administer medication at least 30 minutes before initiating transfusion.	
___	___	___	2. Gather all equipment.	
___	___	___	3. Perform hand hygiene and put on PPE, if indicated.	
___	___	___	4. Identify the patient.	
___	___	___	5. Assemble equipment to the bedside stand or overbed table or other surface within reach.	
___	___	___	6. Close the curtains around the bed and close the door to the room, if possible. Explain what you are going to do and why you are going to do it to the patient. Ask the patient about previous experience with a transfusion and any reactions. Advise the patient to report any chills, itching, rash, or unusual symptoms.	
___	___	___	7. Prime blood administration set with the normal saline IV fluid.	
___	___	___	8. Put on gloves. If the patient does not have a venous access device in place, initiate peripheral venous access. Connect the administration set to the venous access device via the extension tubing. Infuse the normal saline per facility policy.	
___	___	___	9. Obtain blood product from blood bank according to facility policy. Scan the bar codes on blood products if required.	
___	___	___	10. Two registered nurses (or other licensed practitioner [hospital/outpatient setting], or responsible adult [home setting]) compare and validate the following information in the presence of the patient with the medical record, patient identification band (hospital/outpatient setting), and the label of the blood product:	
___	___	___	• Medical order for transfusion of blood product	
___	___	___	• Informed consent	
___	___	___	• Patient identification number	

Excellent	Satisfactory	Needs Practice		Comments
—	—	—	• Patient name	
—	—	—	• Blood group and type	
—	—	—	• Expiration date	
—	—	—	• Inspection of blood product for clots, clumping, gas bubbles	
—	—	—	11. *Obtain baseline set of vital signs before beginning the transfusion.*	
—	—	—	12. Put on gloves. If using an electronic infusion device, put the device on "hold." Close the roller clamp closest to the drip chamber on the saline side of the administration set. Close the roller clamp on the administration set below the infusion device. Alternately, if infusing via gravity, close the roller clamp on the administration set.	
—	—	—	13. Close the roller clamp closest to the drip chamber on the blood product side of the administration set. Remove the protective cap from the access port on the blood container. Remove the cap from the access spike on the administration set. Using a pushing and twisting motion, insert the spike into the access port on the blood container, taking care not to contaminate the spike. Hang the blood container on the IV pole. Open the roller clamp on the blood side of the administration set. Squeeze drip chamber until the in-line filter is saturated. Remove gloves.	
—	—	—	14. *Start administration slowly (approximately 2 mL per minute for the first 15 minutes) (INS, 2016b). Stay with the patient for the first 5 to 15 minutes of transfusion. Open the roller clamp on the administration set below the infusion device. Set the flow rate and begin the transfusion.* Alternately, start the flow of solution by releasing the clamp on the tubing and counting the drops. Adjust until the correct drop rate is achieved. Assess the flow of the blood and function of the infusion device. Inspect the insertion site for signs of infiltration.	
—	—	—	15. Observe the patient for flushing, dyspnea, itching, hives or rash, or any unusual comments.	
—	—	—	16. Reassess vital signs after 15 minutes. Obtain vital signs thereafter according to facility policy and nursing assessment.	
—	—	—	17. After the observation period (5 to 15 minutes) increase the infusion rate to the calculated rate to complete the infusion within the prescribed time frame, no more than 4 hours.	

Excellent	Satisfactory	Needs Practice	SKILL 40-5 **Administering a Blood Transfusion** *(Continued)*	
				Comments
——	——	——	18. Maintain the prescribed flow rate as ordered or as deemed appropriate based on the patient's overall condition, keeping in mind the outer limits for safe administration. Ongoing monitoring is crucial throughout the entire duration of the blood transfusion for early identification of any adverse reactions.	
——	——	——	19. *During transfusion, assess frequently for transfusion reaction. Stop blood transfusion if you suspect a reaction. Quickly replace the blood tubing with a new administration set primed with normal saline for IV infusion. Initiate an infusion of normal saline for IV at an open rate, usually 40 mL/hr. Obtain vital signs. Notify primary care provider and blood bank.*	
——	——	——	20. When transfusion is complete, close the roller clamp on blood side of the administration set and open the roller clamp on the normal saline side of the administration set. Initiate infusion of normal saline. When all of blood has infused into the patient, clamp the administration set. Obtain vital signs. Put on gloves. Cap the access site or resume previous IV infusion. Dispose of blood-transfusion equipment or return to blood bank, according to facility policy.	
——	——	——	21. Remove equipment. Ensure the patient's comfort. Remove gloves. Lower the bed, if not in the lowest position.	
——	——	——	22. Remove additional PPE, if used. Perform hand hygiene.	
——	——	——	23. Monitor and assess the patient after the transfusion for signs and symptoms of delayed transfusion reaction. Provide patient education about signs and symptoms of delayed transfusion reactions.	